Riding the Cancer Coaster: Survival Guide for Teens and Young Adults

Clarissa Schilstra

Copyright © 2015 Clarissa Schilstra

ISBN: 1514208083
ISBN-13: 978-1514208083

"Every teen with cancer, their parents, friends, doctors and nurses should read this book. Clarissa Schilstra writes from profound personal experience in a poignant, clear and no holds barred manner about the psychological implications of undergoing treatment as a teenager. She offers straightforward recommendations for coping and in the process tells those that wish to help how they can be most effective. You won't put it down until you finish."

Stephen Schimpff, MD
Former Director,
University of Maryland
Greenbaum
Cancer Center
and author, Fixing The
Primary Care Crisis

Donald Small, MD, PhD
Director of
Pediatric Oncology,
Sidney Kimmel
Comprehensive
Cancer Center at
Johns Hopkins Hospital

"In *Riding the Cancer Coaster: Survival Guide for Teens and Young Adults* Clarissa Schilstra, a 2-time cancer survivor who went through treatment both as a child and adolescent, has shared her journey and the wisdom she has gained along the way. This inspirational book is a must-read for any teenager or young adult going through cancer therapy as well as for the parents of these patients."

"Clarissa Schilstra offers knowledge, wisdom, and advice to teenagers and young adults who are facing the travails of a cancer diagnosis. Drawing from her own experience, employing plain talk and empathy, she offers helpful suggestions for the entire family. This is an essential book for anyone you know who is going through this life-changing chapter in his or her life."

Paul F. Levy
Former CEO,
Beth Israel
Deaconess
Medical Center

Sharon Perfetti
Co-Founder/
Executive Director
Cool Kids Campaign

"Pediatric cancer is something that can only be understood by those who have lived through it. Clarissa is able to offer readers the extremely unique perspective of having survived two bouts of cancer before she even turned 16. Therefore, her advice and insight is sound and a must read for both patients and caregivers."

"Twenty-nine years ago, I was diagnosed with leukemia. No one in my family, nor any of my friends, had suffered this diagnosis. I didn't even know at the time that leukemia was a form of cancer. This was before the Internet, so I couldn't 'google' it. There were very few survivor support groups, because there were very few survivors of leukemia in 1986. And the doctors guessed that I had eighteen months to live. No one had written a book like this one by Clarissa Schilstra to tell the story, to tell people what to expect, and to help survivors understand and cope with what they were about to experience. Leukemia is not like a broken arm; no one sees it but you know it is there every day. Clarissa tells it like it is - nausea, burning headaches, hair loss, friend loss, time loss, and fear. But she does it in the most positive way for all survivors and their families to read, and learn, and use. The lessons she shares were hard learned, but Clarissa's book can help survivors cope with medicine, doctors, family and friends; with fears and challenges; and with living with cancer, not dying from it. I have been through the battle with leukemia and bladder cancer, and I wish Clarissa's book had been around for me to read - and for my family to read – twenty-nine years ago. Thank you, Clarissa."

Mark H. Kolman
Two-time cancer survivor

DEDICATION

To my little brother Erik, for being my best friend through it all.

CONTENTS

ACKNOWLEDGMENTS

Stephen Schimpff, MD
For his support, guidance, and assistance throughout
the last few years, as I developed my blog and this book

Paul and Christina Schilstra
My amazing parents who have been there for me always and
encouraged me to make this book happen

Lori Wiener, PhD, DCSW, FAPOS
For her contribution to this book and
her willingness to provide advice

The doctors, nurses, and staff of Johns Hopkins Pediatric Oncology,
especially my nurse Sue Rodgers
For your amazing care, ever-present smiles, and dedication to your patients
- I would not have survived without your expert care and compassion

FOREWORD

Lori Wiener, PhD, DCSW, FAPOS

Riding the Cancer Coaster: Survival Guide for Teens and Young Adults offers insights to teens and young adults whose lives have been touched with cancer and to their family members and medical providers who care for them. Clarissa Schilstra takes each reader through the journey of her cancer experience, from what she remembers from her diagnosis and treatment of leukemia at the age of two and a half, her life as a healthy child, and the devastation of disease recurrence ten years later, at the age of thirteen. While Clarissa talks about how her life has been turned upside down, she provides a tool for teens to learn how they can navigate the psychological and social impact of childhood cancer and cope with medication side effects and toxicities along with the physical and emotional changes that follow.

Clarissa was able to describe many of the critical events and emotional responses present at diagnosis ("...the surreal feeling of waking up in a hospital bed day after day, hooked up to a million things, and wondering what you did to get there in the first place"); during the initiation and continuation of treatment (dealing with adverse effects, including hair loss, weight changes, psychological adaption); isolation ("It is like I am in this little boat all alone in the middle of this vast ocean. It is like I'm in this little rowboat, doing everything I can to survive, while everyone else my age is on this giant cruise ship right next to me, having fun and enjoying life. It is right there next to me so I can see it and hear about it, but I can never reach it."); and the new challenges that accompany end of treatment and survivorship (changing priorities, peer acceptance, neurocognitive changes, questions of fertility). Fear of recurrence and its intense redefining of all the issues youth experience throughout treatment represent a further challenge for patients and families. Clarissa does a beautiful job bringing these to light.

While Clarissa eloquently describes the invisible psychological impact that cancer treatment can have on a young person, the sections that most clearly illustrate her insight are on the impact on one's family and friends. For example, she wrote: "I think it is important for others to remember that, in that moment, you are not only thinking of your own world, you are thinking of how this will affect your friends and family." Clarissa resonated with the words of Hazel Grace from the book and movie, *The Fault in Our Stars*, "I could not let the grenade that was my body detonate and leave their world completely obliterated. I was determined not to let that happen." Even after treatment ends, Clarissa reminds the reader that the psychological impact does not end - for themselves or for their family members. "I had completely forgotten that my mom and dad might not find it so easy to bounce back. So, when going through this post-treatment transition, keep in mind your parents and family members are transitioning too."

The tremendous impact that childhood cancer can have on healthy siblings is worthy of a book in itself. Clarissa brought this to life with a powerful quote from her younger brother. "I felt like the only child of divorced parents." Clarissa recognized how the family separation caused by her treatment affected him. To others who have a brother or sister affected by their disease, she recommends, " It is a great idea to try and have some "normal" time with your siblings. Play a game with them, take time to hang out and talk, or watch a movie together."

In terms of the struggle that so many experience due to feeling disconnected from their social network, Clarissa wrote, "Sometimes it is necessary to tell your friends you want them to let you know if they are getting together and that you will make the decision if you are well enough to come along, or not." She does not shy away from the pain of losing friends. "Many of these teens are or were my friends. I cannot help but wonder why. I get angry, I cry, I pray, I hope, I hurt. While my first confrontation with mortality left me feeling guilty and frustrated, these others leave me with yet another host of feelings: heartbreak, terror, and inspiration all interwoven together." Yet throughout the book, Clarissa provides readers with a message of hope and the importance of finding one's inner strength. She writes, " Relish the fact that you have a chance to showcase your perseverance. Do not hang your head in shame for having no hair. And realize, that one day in the not so distant future, you may actually miss that bald head of yours and all that it represented." These examples exemplify the resilience that many children and families demonstrate when facing cancer during their teen and young adult lives and the remarkable human capacity to adjust, and even flourish in the face of disease recurrence.

Clarissa was fortunate to have state-of-the-art care, an exceptionally supportive family who were strong advocates for her medical and emotional needs, and she remains disease free. Yet, there is also the reality that unequal treatment and availability of psychosocial care remain problems in cancer care throughout the world. While everyone's experiences will differ, there is clearly useful and inspiriting information in *Riding the Cancer Coaster: Survival Guide for Teens and Young Adults* for anyone touched by cancer.

INTRODUCTION

When I was thirteen, after ten years of living disease-free, I had a relapse of acute lymphoblastic leukemia. My prognosis was poor – I had a forty percent chance of survival.

Being thirteen as opposed to two and a half years old, I was entirely conscious of the trials I would face. As much as I am a proponent of positivity and humor, that moment was the most serious moment of my entire life. I knew, lying on the operating room table, hearing the words of my oncologist, listening to him as he caught his breath from running all the way from the eighth floor Pediatric Oncology clinic to the basement of the surgical floor, watching him as he told us the news, registering the words he spoke as he told me my chance of living through this was only forty percent...I knew this would be an experience that would define the rest of my life. The moment I looked over at my sobbing parents, I knew my life would never be the same.

Most people tend to write memoirs at the end of their lives, to reflect on lessons and experiences, usually because a person does not learn lessons or have seriously significant experiences until he or she has gone through a large portion of his or her life. In my case, it has been much different. My "adventures" began the moment I entered the world, and continue as I write these words. In my twenty-one years of life so far, I have lived through a lot. In many ways, that has been a blessing and in other ways it has been an enormous struggle.

My struggles began when I was born, unexpectedly eleven weeks early. I was only three pounds at birth. My parents waited anxiously through my first week of life, watching me through the clear box they call an isolette, until I was declared a feeder-grower. Sure enough, they fed me and I grew.

When I was two and a half years old, I was diagnosed with acute lymphoblastic leukemia for the first time. Aside from various complications with my port-a-cath failing, contracting Respiratory Syncytial Virus, ending up with a bit of a hard time walking because of the Vincristine chemotherapy I was receiving, and having all of this go on with a six month old baby brother at home, my family and I survived with flying colors. I do not remember much from those years.

I would have had a fairly healthy childhood after that initial cancer experience had I not almost blinded myself by accidentally putting a hole in my cornea at ten years old, with the spackle knife I was using to help my parents strip wall paper in our bathroom. I apparently missed my pupil by less than a millimeter. Thanks to that stroke of luck, an incredible eye surgeon, and four tiny stitches, I regained the excellent vision I had before the accident.

Because the majority of my post-cancer childhood was full of amazing travels with my family, good friends, and academic achievements of which I was so proud, my parents and I were convinced I was done with my traumatic health scares.

1

But, only two years after nearly blinding myself, just before my thirteenth birthday, I found out my leukemia had relapsed. What was worse, the leukemia had not only relapsed in my bloodstream, but it had formed in my spinal fluid as well. That was when, against my will, I had to jump on the cancer roller coaster and endure two and half years of chemotherapy and radiation. Normally, roller coasters are fun and you choose to ride them. You know the ride will end in a few minutes and you will likely walk away with a smile on your face. The cancer coaster is something else entirely. You have no choice but to get on, there is no certainty of a happy ending, and you have no idea how or when it will end. You may find yourself alive or dead at the end of the ride, but you have to get on anyway. It takes you to heights you never dreamed of and to lows of unspeakable horrors.

It is estimated that, globally, about 173,000 adolescents and young adults are diagnosed with cancer each year (Cancer Research UK, 2008[1]). That means at least 173,000 young people and their families must ride the cancer coaster each year, with no control over what happens to them in the process.

Although the physical impact of cancer treatment is severe and visible, I found that the psychological impact is just as severe, but often invisible. As a teenager or young adult, you strive for independence, but cancer leaves you completely dependent on everyone around you. During an age when you are obsessed with your appearance, you find yourself without a hair on your head or body. Due to a completely compromised immune system, isolation leaves you starving for social contact. When you should be able to start looking forward and setting goals for the future, your dreams are put on hold. Our emotions are already difficult to control, but the trauma of cancer tips the balance and can make staying positive very difficult. Personally, I had a great deal of trouble finding other teenage girls going through a similar cancer treatment at the same time as I was, leaving me struggling to find someone who could grasp the gravity of what I was going through. I also could not find any resources for someone my age, to help me through the social and emotional challenges I was facing.

That is how I arrived here. The idea for this book arose from that struggle to understand what I was feeling, what I was going through, and how I was going to live through it. As a combination of a memoir and self-help book, I hope that, through these pages, I can provide a resource to teens and young adults with cancer. It is also my hope that it can serve as a source of support for anyone going through any kind of significant health experience.

I do not claim to be an expert, especially since I am only just entering my final year of college. But, I have experience, which I have reflected on for years, and carefully reviewed to be able to put it into words so that it can be useful to others. I do not guarantee that any of my recommendations will be successful, but it is my goal to give you at least a place to start, when learning to cope with the ups and downs of your cancer coaster ride. For additional resources and articles, you can also check out my blog at www.teen-cancer.com.

1 THE BEGINNING OF IT ALL

As Julie Andrews once sang in *The Sound of Music*, "Let's start at the very beginning, a very good place to start."

Some of my earliest memories are of my first journey through cancer treatment. I remember the sounds of the playroom and the cherry smell they put into the mask I was given for anesthesia before spinal taps. I remember the empty plastic syringe my nurse gave me so I could play doctor on my dolls. I remember being about four years old and knowing exactly how to set up my dolls with an IV: numbing cream first, arm board second, fake needle in, tape on, connect syringe, open the clamp on the tubes, and push.

Fortunately, I only have those few memories from that time. I simply know that I successfully completed my treatment and went on to have an absolutely wonderful childhood. Although I was under the impression the rest of my life would be entirely healthy, my cancer relapsed ten years after my first diagnosis, when I was thirteen years old. It was the summer before eighth grade and my life changed drastically. I came to understand what feeling "sick and tired" really meant.

Feeling Powerless

For me, one of the hardest parts of hearing the news was not the news itself, but the feeling of being powerless. When I was diagnosed with the relapse, I was lying on an operating room table. I was about to be put under anesthesia, in order to have a diagnostic spinal tap and bone marrow aspiration and so the doctors could find out more about what was wrong with me.

A spinal tap, also known as a lumbar puncture, is a procedure in which a sample of cerebrospinal fluid is taken, via a needle, from your spinal column. A bone marrow aspiration is a procedure in which a sample of bone marrow, the soft tissue inside of your bones, is obtained by inserting a needle into a bone (typically mine were performed on my hip bone).

My parents were standing across from the bed I was on, since they had been waiting for me to go under. The anesthesiologist had his finger on the syringe and was just about to push, when the pediatric oncologist came running in. He said the words that blew my world apart: "It's leukemia."

Considering my previous history, my parents knew what that meant. That moment is as crystal clear in my memory today, as it will be, no doubt, forever. While my parents knew what was coming, I did not remember enough from my first bout with cancer to have an idea of what to expect. All I could think about was that I had to relinquish control of my life to another human being – the doctor – who I had only met the day before. I did not understand what "forty percent chance of survival" really meant either – I was a teenager with a life to live; I did not grasp the possibility that my life might be taken away from me. Yet, I was forced to place all of my trust in that doctor.

The shock and disbelief I felt upon hearing my diagnosis was soon followed by a feeling of bizarre clarity. It was as if some sort of survival mechanism kicked in and told me to get ready to do whatever it would take, before I could even think about being scared. Now, I think that clarity actually came from the fact my brain could not comprehend that such an illness could actually kill me. I guess I still had enough of a sense of teenage invincibility to keep myself contently in denial that I had a life-threatening illness.

Aside from my own feelings and thoughts, what I remember most of all was looking over at my parents as they fell apart. I was more worried about making this okay for them than I was worried about myself. As Hazel Grace so eloquently referred to it in *The Fault in Our Stars*[2] movie, I could not let the grenade that was my body detonate and leave their world completely obliterated. I was determined not to let that happen.

In some way, I think it is important for others to remember that, in the moment of diagnosis, you are not only thinking of your own world, you are thinking of how this will affect your friends and family.

Life, as you know it, suddenly stops, and you are left to wonder if it is all real. All that ran through my head during the following hours was: "Could this really be happening to me?"

It all became very real, however, when my first chemotherapy started on the night of my diagnosis. That is when I got scared. Seeing the treatment happening, feeling its initial impact on me, and learning about the road I was about to travel down led my mind to finally recognize I was actually in danger. There was a chance I might not survive, that my treatment might not work, and that was terrifying. I became angry at the same time because it just seemed so unfair, so random, and so devastating. The sense of loss was greatest though because I soon learned of the amount of time I would have to spend in the hospital, of the school I would miss, and of the uncertainty of my future. I grieved for the impending loss of two and a half years of my "normal" teenage life.

Looking back, I definitely think I put on too much of a stoic face and kind of swept all my feelings under a rug. I guess I just tried to ignore the fact that my prognosis was not good, that I might not survive, and that I would have to spend the next two years going through some very uncomfortable things. Granted, this was an effective survival mechanism at the time, but it was probably not the healthiest choice for the long-term. I did not allow myself to outwardly express those emotions. So, now that I am six years cancer free, I think I still have a sense of fear and uncertainty on a daily basis, manifesting itself as impatience, anxiety, and being risk averse, because I never learned to experience and move past those emotions at the very beginning. Therefore, to help save you from that same experience, here are my suggestions.

What to do with the shock, fear, worry, and uncertainty:
In retrospect, I definitely think it is more important that you allow yourself time to experience your emotions. You should take it slow so that you can find a way to understand and move beyond them, such that they do not plague you down the line. To save you from the mistakes I made, here are my suggestions.

Step 1: Talk. Talking about those feelings is a great release. If possible, turn to your friends and family for support. You should definitely try talking about what you are going through, and your parents or those in your immediate support system should make sure that you are talking and not keeping your emotions quietly tucked away. You can also talk with your doctors and nurses, or a mental health care provider. There is a field dedicated to the mental health of people living with cancer, called psycho-oncology, and psycho-oncologists can help you cope with the social, emotional, and spiritual effects of the cancer experience.

After a few weeks of getting to know my outpatient nurse, she became my new best friend and was a huge support to me. She was very good at talking with me and encouraging me, sharing her years of pediatric oncology experience to bring me hope. Talking with her calmed my fears, subdued my anger, and gave me something positive to focus on instead of the sense of loss that would otherwise have dragged me down.

Long story short, you have to let your emotions out if you are going to stay sane and not become depressed or anxious. Being diagnosed with cancer, or any serious illness for that matter, is one of the most surreal experiences a person can go through. For me, it felt like I was in a nightmare and I could not wake up. Other teens I have talked to say that it felt as if a truck ran them over, backed up, and ran them over again.

That brings us to the next challenge after diagnosis: the surreal feeling of waking up in a hospital bed day after day, hooked up to a million things, and wondering what you did to get there in the first place.

Step 2: Accept it. I know, for me, it took months to accept cancer as the new reality of my life and to move forward. Cancer treatment begins incredibly quickly, and that speed in itself can be scary and extremely difficult to handle. The fact you are transitioning from your normal life and comfortable world into an incredibly uncomfortable and scary place just compounds the problem. Questioning the reality of the situation, and wondering if you are dreaming, is normal. Feeling pain and anguish is normal. It takes time before you "wake up" and are able to realize this is your new reality. Let's face it, when you are thrown into a hospital and given all kinds of medications the day after you are diagnosed, it is difficult to process everything that has happened. You are thrown into this foreign world, this painful life, within moments. Try to give yourself time to accept it all. Unfortunately, I did not find any particular way to expedite this acclimating process, it just takes some time.

Once the chaos has settled, the next challenge that usually comes along is dealing with the sudden transition from normal life to hospital life.

<u>Step 3</u>: Pack the essentials. When admitted into the hospital, bring your favorite pillows, blankets, movies, games, or anything from home that helps you (blankie included, if you are like me and need something to comfort you! Seriously!). These things can help you feel a little more comfortable in the new environment. Filling your hospital room with your belongings from home and decorating it in fun, unique ways can liven up the room and make it visually interesting and physically comforting. One of my favorite room decorations was the card chain my mom made for me. She collected all of the cards I received from friends and family, punched holes in them, and tied them all to a ribbon so we could bring them along and hang them on the wall to brighten up my hospital room each time I had an inpatient stay. A friend of mine, who also went through cancer treatment as a teenager, said she liked to put up wall or window clings, as well as printed pictures. She found they made for great talking points when people came to visit or when the doctors stopped in. More importantly, they helped distract her from chemo by reminding her of all of the fun things she was fighting to get back to.

2 GETTING THROUGH THE MEDICAL LOOPS

Waking up the morning after my relapse diagnosis, to the beeping of my IV pole, and opening my eyes to the bag of pinkish toxin already dripping into my chest through the newly installed metal port-a-cath sticking up just below my skin's surface, was awful. It was the first slip into a downhill ride that took me through many loops of medical challenges. While you will face many ups and downs throughout your treatment, you may find the most complicated are the medical loops – the medical obstacles about which you may not have been warned. In order to help you remain on as smooth of a course as possible, it is important you understand what to expect from such medical loops. Therefore, I want to take some time to talk about all the medical things that those amazing medical people do not tell you enough about. Some of these challenges are what my mom likes to refer to as the "tangent" issues, the ones that oncologists often do not handle well since their primary focus is eliminating the cancer.

Nausea

The first challenge you will likely encounter after your diagnosis is nausea. While your care team has likely warned you about this side effect that is universally associated with chemotherapy and cancer treatment, it sucks nonetheless. However, nowadays there are actually quite a few ways to combat it. I suggest, above all, that you remember the names of the medications they give you for nausea so that you can keep track of what works and what does not. You may find it easier to remember the medicines you have been taking by keeping a medication log, either by typing or writing down the medications you take. This will be crucial because you will have to know what you want when the new concoctions of chemotherapy they give you make any flu-related nausea you may have previously experienced seem like a vacation in comparison.

To get you started, here are my favorite contenders in the battle against nausea: Zofran, Ativan, Zantac, Benadryl, and above all, Emend. Zofran (also known as Ondansetron) is an anti-nausea medicine that was designed for chemotherapy nausea. It worked very well for me, but is not effective for everyone, so be sure to ask your healthcare team if you want other options.

Benadryl is the well-known allergy medicine that you have likely taken in the past. However, when given intravenously, it can send you off to a deep slumber and away from all of that discomfort. It is especially handy because it can be used along with Zofran and other preferred anti-nausea medicines.

Then, we have Ativan (also known as Lorazepam). Ativan is actually an anti-anxiety medicine, but it can be very effective when used in conjunction with another anti-nausea medicine because it really relaxes you, which somehow seems to be effective in combating nausea.

With both Ativan and Benadryl, you can also request just a half dose if you are not looking to pass out or pee in your pants (which will not necessarily happen on a full dose, that was just the case for me!).

Next, we have Zantac, which is an over-the-counter medicine to treat conditions that cause the stomach to produce more acid than usual. This can happen with chemotherapy, so while Zantac does not necessarily help with nausea directly, it can help your stomach to stay a little more balanced.

Finally, we have the invention from heaven that seriously saved my life while going through my treatment: Emend (Aprepitant). Emend had only just been approved by the U.S. government's Food and Drug Administration (FDA) for use by adults when I began my treatment. After many failed attempts to control my nausea during those first few weeks of incredibly intense chemotherapy, one of my doctors recommended we look into it. Although I was only thirteen, I was the size and weight of an adult. Therefore, after some discussion and paperwork, I was approved to begin Emend.

Perhaps the best example of the effectiveness of this miracle medicine was how it helped me during my methotrexate weekends. For those of you who are not familiar with the dandelion yellow poison that is methotrexate, it is a very effective chemotherapy for leukemia patients. However, I received it over a twenty-four hour period, as in "we are going to let a glass bottle of neon yellow toxin, about the size of a liter of soda, drip into you over twenty-four hours."

They then flush it out of you over the next two to three days by hanging about four times as much fluid, and forcing you to pee every two hours. They do not let you leave the hospital until the methotrexate level in your bloodstream is down to a certain level. That, of course requires a lot of output if you know what I mean. It takes a really long time to get the methotrexate level down if the only thing flushing your system is IV fluid – meaning you are just peeing. Really, it takes some eating so you can get rid of it the other way too. Unfortunately, methotrexate given over twenty-four hours does not exactly leave one feeling hungry. So, my typical methotrexate hospital stays were at least five days long.

Then, Emend came along. Not only did it make it possible for me to eat after the infusion, but it actually enabled me to eat <u>during</u> the infusion. That translated into more output and less methotrexate in my blood stream. So, my five-day stays went down to three-day stays. That meant I had a chance at almost a full week at home in between those inpatient stays. Those extra days at home gave my family some more time to be together.

Spinal Taps, Pain, and Paying Attention
Other than nausea, chemotherapy and the many other parts of treatment can cause a host of challenging side effects. One of the worst experiences I ever had in my life was all because of a spinal tap, a spinal tap that happened the second week of my relapse treatment.

Leukemia patients receive anywhere from fifteen to twenty spinal taps throughout their treatment. That meant that before I had even begun my relapse treatment, I had scarring in my back from the nineteen spinal taps I had during my treatment as a child. Spinal taps can only happen in a very small region in your lower back, so due to my leukemia history it was difficult for them to access my spinal fluid from the usual location. This caused serious challenges when one of the physician assistants, one who had likely performed thousands of spinal taps in her career, took numerous tries to get into my spinal fluid. Thank heavens I was under anesthesia. Anyway, after the procedure, I went into the recovery room afterward, as usual. Then, I was wheeled back to the inpatient floor and went home later that day.

The next morning, I woke up with a headache. It was not a normal headache, as it was in the very front and center of my forehead and came with a pounding pain. Instead of feeling better as the days went by, I felt worse and worse. There came a point when I could not even sit up anymore. I had to lie down to achieve relief and keep myself from vomiting from the pain.

At my next clinic appointment, a week later, I was visibly in pain and could not remain sitting up while I met with the doctor (to note: he was just the clinic doctor for the day, not my doctor). He explained to me that I was having what was called a spinal headache, and it was a fairly common after-effect of spinal taps. It is caused by spinal fluid leaking out, resulting in a depletion of the spinal fluid that is supposed to surround the brain and essentially keep it padded within your skull. Spinal headaches are supposed to heal after a short time though, so I was sent home and given some extra oxycodone for my pain. After two days of the pain becoming ever more excruciating, my mom contacted the doctor on-call and explained my situation, inquiring if there was anything else they could do for my unrelenting pain. The doctor prescribed me caffeine pills, which were supposed to help constrict my blood vessels and make it easier for my back to heal and stop the leak. Those of course did nothing; they did not even help me think more clearly. My chemotherapy treatment continued.

In spite of all the pain I was experiencing because of my headache, one of my favorite moments from my entire treatment happened on the day of my next bone marrow aspiration. My amazing doctor was there to do the aspiration. He knew I was in a lot of pain, so as I lay on the stretcher, after leaving my parents to go to the operating room, he held my hand and smiled at me. Suddenly, I felt like someone was determined to save me and I knew I would survive. I knew this guy was going to help me get better and it was awesome.

My dad then did research on how to fix spinal leaks. He found out about a procedure called an epidural blood patch. In such a procedure, blood is taken from a vein in the arm and injected into the area of the spinal column where the hole is. The blood then clots and seals the hole. The problem was, when we presented the idea to my doctors, they said we could not do it. Why, you may ask, was this not possible?

Cancer, the stupid cancer that landed me with that headache, was the problem. During the first two weeks of my spinal headache, I was not yet in remission (they were not sure the cancer was gone from my blood), so they could not take blood from my arm and put it in my spinal column. They had just determined that all the leukemia in my spinal fluid was gone and did not want to put the leukemia from my blood stream back into my nice, clean spinal fluid. So, we waited.

The days continued to go by until the blessed day when I was at my usual outpatient appointment and my doctor came in to tell me I was in remission. There was no longer any leukemia visible in my spinal column or my blood. I was on my way to beating my forty percent chance of survival.

I was also on my way for more treatment. The chemotherapy continued and I continued to lose weight, while the pain became more and more unbearable. At the end of the twenty-six days of agonizing head pain, so blinding that it made it impossible for me to eat or even use the bathroom without vomiting, my mom turned on her mama bear mode and called the clinic and told them, "My daughter is dying and I need you to do something now! She won't be here to treat if you don't fix this spinal headache."

She got approval to take me to the ER. I laid on a sleeping bag in the back of our minivan because I could not sit up in the car seat. When we got to the ER, they came out with a stretcher, which my mom had demanded be there upon our arrival. They wheeled me in and gave me the well-known question of "rate your pain on a scale of one to ten." Stupid me tried to smile still and I was like, "probably nine." (Hint: you should not be like nice Clarissa when you want people to fix a problem for you. You have to be honest, and I do not know why I was not). Really, it was 9,000 on a scale of one to ten. I was then admitted to the oncology floor and my mom got really angry with the doctors during rounds (the term used to describe the doctors' daily visits to patients' rooms around the inpatient unit) the next day. My doctor was not present for those rounds since he was not on inpatient duty.

I initially hated her for going rogue on a group of well-meaning physicians like that, but now I realize she was doing her job and protecting me. It worked too, because I was taken to the CT scanner at three o'clock in the morning to have a scan of my back done. They were finally going to try and see what could be prolonging my spinal headache pain. It turned out I had more than a little leak; I had a serious hole in the fluid column that was not able to heal because of the chemotherapy that had been injected into my spinal fluid. This was great to know but not helpful in relieving my pain.

After waiting one more day for them to coordinate the necessary procedure, I was on my way to the pain clinic to get my epidural blood patch. That was a literal miracle. I had not been a human being for twenty-eight days, lost in a sea of agonizing pain. I had lost twenty-five pounds in less than four weeks. But, the minute that anesthesiologist took blood from my arm and injected it into the very spot where my leak originated, the pain stopped. It just stopped. Within three hours, I could think and see and feel clearly once again. It was incredible.

So, you may wonder why I tell you this story in such detail. Well, it is for several reasons. First, it is to advise you to always be honest about how you are feeling, and to not put on a brave face when you want or need something to be done. If you are in pain, tell the providers honestly about your pain.

Second, fight for what you want or step aside and let your parents, or someone else in your support system, fight for you. By stepping aside, my mom could make sure that something would be done for me.

Third of all, pay attention. Doctors are trained in medicine, but they are not gods. They can make mistakes and they can miss things. Sometimes you have to find your own answers and push them to listen. You may want to consult doctors from other specialties, such as palliative care doctors, who can help address physical and emotional pain. The Internet is also great source, although you should certainly exercise caution when using the Internet for resources since not all websites are credible. The sites listed at the end of this book are all credible resources that address a variety of cancer treatment-related issues.

Last, but not least, look for the miracles in the midst of your worst moments. Those painful days were the worst of my life. But, it was during them that I saw the greatest compassion in the face of a young physician, who gave me such hope.

Allergic Reactions

Another important issue to be aware of is allergic reactions. To me, they were like a plague: rarely seen but fierce and scary when they occur. When you are someone like me, however, all things rare occur (fun fact: there was less than a one percent chance my cancer would come back after being in remission for ten years, but it happened anyway). So, I have had my fair share of allergic reactions.

Here are my experiences with reactions. In describing all of this, my hope is that you are able to become aware of potential risks and know that there are often alternative options to help you minimize uncomfortable reactions. I never knew that any platelets or chemotherapies could cause me to stop breathing. They do not usually warn patients about things that are "unlikely" to happen. But you may be one of those "unlikely" patients and I guess they just do not like to tell you about reactions that rarely occur. So, I am telling you now!

First, there are blood products. Before receiving any blood transfusions, you may be given Tylenol and Benadryl, or some related mixture, to help prevent your body from reacting to the foreign matter that is needed to keep you alive. Usually, this mixture of medicine works. However, in my case, I had some other problems.

Because of my spinal headache, I had been lying down constantly for an extended period of time. Combine that with platelet infusions (to combat the reducing platelet count that resulted from my chemotherapies) and the clotting tendencies of the birth control I was given (to prevent me from menstruating while on chemotherapy) and I ended up with a nice big blood clot in the iliac vein (big, main vein) of my hip. They called it a deep-vein thrombosis.

So, I was started on anti-clotting injections. It is important to note that treatment for blood clots thins your blood and makes you prone to bleeding. Lower platelet counts also make you prone to bleeding. A battle of balance ensued between giving me more platelets to keep my platelet count at a reasonable level, and giving me enough medication to get rid of my blood clot.

Therefore, I received more and more platelet infusions, until I had my first allergic reaction: hives. Oh, the itching! It was awful. The platelet infusion was immediately stopped and I was given more antihistamines as well as epinephrine (a drug commonly used to help stop the symptoms of serious allergic reactions – it is the same as the medication in an EpiPen, if you are more familiar with that). Eventually, the itching calmed down.

For my next transfusions, I was carefully monitored. Then, I reacted again after receiving a bag of platelets. This, however, was more serious than the last because I spiked a high fever, during which I began to hallucinate. They tried Tylenol and other fever-reducing medicines, but nothing worked and my temperature continued to increase, reaching 104.5 degrees at its peak. That was when they went old school and covered me in a tarp and then poured piles of ice all over me. I will never forget that feeling, wanting nothing more than to pile more and more blankets on myself to get warm, but instead being covered in ice that made me even more freezing than my fever chills did. But, the ice worked and I eventually cooled down.

It was soon determined that I needed to have my platelets "spun" the next time I receive them, which means most of the donor plasma is removed from around the platelets to decrease the amount of material against which your body would react. This helped for a while, until I once again had a reaction.

This time I had the most feared reaction: anaphylaxis. To put that more simply, I could not breathe. It felt as if my lungs were being squeezed and my throat was closing in and honestly it was the most terrifying feeling I have ever had. That reaction brought in an avalanche of nurses and doctors. Oxygen mask went on, epinephrine went in, pulse monitor went on, I mean it was straight out of Grey's Anatomy. So, from then on my platelets were both spun and washed, which means they spun them and then used saline to rinse off any donor material that might be on the cells. This finally worked and I had no more reactions to platelets.

However, that was the mere beginning of my reaction woes. I developed a serious full-body rash after receiving an intravenous antibiotic called Vancomycin. I was put on the Vancomycin after developing an infection in the area of my thigh where I had received PEG-Asparaginase chemotherapy injections.

The day after I received the shots, a red welt began forming on my right thigh, around the injection site. I was given some ice and it was monitored, but it kept growing larger and warmer. I could barely walk on that leg because it caused so much pain in my muscle.

At the worst point, it became so warm and red you could probably have fried an egg on it. Then, they began to worry, and it was determined that an infection had likely developed. So, I was placed on the Vancomycin. However, the Vancomycin could only be given intravenously and needed to be done over a two-week period. The Vancomycin seemed to be helping my leg. Unfortunately, close to the end of the second week, I started itching all over and became incredibly hot. That was when the weird, red, and splotchy rash happened. Sadly for me and my hot and itchy self, it was determined that the reaction was not serious enough to stop the antibiotics, so I was just given some Benadryl, which calmed my system down.

I faced anaphylaxis reactions two more times due to chemotherapies. The first was a reaction to the PEG-Asparaginase (I guess maybe, after that infection on my thigh, my body did not want any more PEG). I was so excited because I had just learned that Johns Hopkins had gotten the intravenous form of PEG, which meant I would no longer need those awful intramuscular injections. My doctors also thought using the intravenous form would help me avoid an infection forming like the last time. So, I said sign me right up! The pump was on and I was all hooked up, but no more than five or ten minutes later, I could not breathe and the usual anaphylaxis drill occurred. Once I was stabilized, the doctor came in and told me it would not be safe to give me PEG anymore.

However, seeing as it was crucial in my fight against the leukemia, something else had to replace it. So, he informed me that I would receive a drug called Erwinia Asparaginase, which was shown in clinical trials to be as effective as PEG but with a different chemical makeup such that I would not likely react to it. Sadly for me, that was only available in an injection form, so back to those thigh shots I went. That being said, I never reacted to Erwinia, so as long as I could breathe freely I was perfectly happy with injections.

The second anaphylactic reaction was a reaction to a chemotherapy called Etoposide, which I received many times. I was having my usual afternoon-long infusion that began with a chemotherapy called Cyclophosphamide and was followed by Etoposide. I had made it through the nauseous morning of Cyclophosphamide, but not long after the Etoposide started, things got ugly. I was just lying there watching Friends on the TV, as I always did, when my lungs became tight and my body was overcome by a warm sensation. Suddenly, I could not breathe and I felt as if I was drowning on the inside. Once again, the alert went up and the monitors went on. After the epinephrine and oxygen mask, I was able to breathe again.

So, allergic reactions can come in many forms and at very unexpected times. Be aware that everyone reacts differently, and that you may not experience any allergic reactions at all. I believe it is better to know they are possible and to understand what they involve, such that you do not think your treatment is killing you, or that you are dying (as I thought I was), the first time you have a serious allergic reaction. Most importantly, the SECOND you experience any type of allergic reaction such as difficulty breathing or itching, call the nurse IMMEDIATELY. Do not wait even a single minute. Those allergic reactions can be very dangerous.

Steroids

Most associate the word steroids with sports scandals and performance enhancement, but I associate them with eating entire pizzas, peeing a lot, and not being able to sleep. The steroids used in cancer treatment are typically corticosteroids, a different kind of steroid than the more popularly known anabolic steroids used in athletic performance enhancement. For those of you who are on any kind of steroids as part of your cancer treatment, whether it is Prednisone, Dexamethasone, or something else, you will become very familiar with their lovely side effects.

For me, Prednisone was not very problematic; I just developed the face of a chipmunk and ate a lot. My real struggles came when I began Dexamethasone. I do not know why, but that was a very different experience. On Dexamethasone, I often had insomnia, I was always thirsty, and I could never get full. One evening, I ate an entire pizza, literally eight slices of pizza, all by myself. Now, my parents only permitted this binge eating because I had not eaten anything at all really during the last few months, because of the intensity of the chemotherapies I was on.

Although my insatiable appetite was certainly a nuisance, and I was not a fan of looking like a swollen blob (steroids make you retain a lot of water), the worst part was really the mood swings. I went from feeling raging anger one minute to feeling exhilarated the next, and then I would all of a sudden want to cry.

For severe steroid-induced mood swings, you can ask to consult with a psychiatrist, since psychiatrists have various tools they can use to provide you some relief. In terms of coping with the physical symptoms induced by steroids, I found that drinking enough water to stay hydrated, but not too much such that I would feel bloated, was helpful. I also tried to limit the quantity of food I was eating to normal portions, and that was useful in helping me to keep my weight gain a bit under control.

Pills

I think a really funny part of going through cancer treatment is the colorful pharmacy you develop in your kitchen cabinet. From pink tablets, to white horse pills, to yellow capsules you may find yourself with pills from all colors of the rainbow. I also found the sheer quantity of pills was humorous. Within three weeks of starting my treatment, my pill bottles had to be relocated to their own basket because they were overtaking our family medicine cabinet.

You should become very familiar with the medicines you take, such that when the new night nurse on the inpatient floor tries to give you your morning pills after your dinner, you will know to – forcefully – tell her "I don't take my fluconazole now, I take that in the morning…and where is my Bactrim? I take that now and not in the morning! Also, I just ate some dinner so can I have my 6MP in like three hours instead of right now?"

But seriously, be on your game or you will find yourself taking all the right medicines at the wrong times, especially at home. As I said about the doctors I will say about the nurses: everyone has your best interests at heart and wants to help, but mistakes will still happen. I love all of the nurses I had but during the first few months, there were definitely a couple of times where that conversation happened.

Make sure to ask questions like:

- Does this medicine have to be given on an empty stomach or with some food?
- Can these two drugs be taken at the same time?
- Do I need to take all thirty-two of my methotrexate pills at the same time or within a certain timeframe?

Ask all the questions you can think of to ensure you are taking your medicines correctly. To this day, my mother believes my relapse was caused by not taking 6MP on an empty stomach during the first six months of my first leukemia treatment. Don't let a medication mistake affect your outcome.

Medication compliance is critical to the success of your treatment!

Shots at Home

I struggled greatly with at-home injections. While I became quite the professional pill-swallower and could handle all sizes of needles, I could never give myself a shot at home. If you can master that skill, more power to you! I opted to have my mom give them to me.

The two medicines I took at home that had to be given as sub-cutaneous shots (i.e. small needle) were the Lovenox shots to treat my blood clot and the GCSF shots that helped me increase my white blood cell count after serious inpatient chemotherapy. Lovenox shots, if you ever have to have them, are a little painful going in because the medicine can sting a bit. But, I found that icing the area a little after the shot or putting some numbing cream on beforehand can help. GCSF, however, was not painful going in but rather caused some serious aching once it started working. If you are put on GCSF and find yourself with joint pain, try walking around and alternating between squatting and standing for a short time. I found those activities helped to decrease the throbbing pain it caused in my joints following the injection.

Masks

Other than the mountains of medications and side effects with which you will become familiar, there is the infamous protective accessory that you will grow to hate: the mask. Rarely coming in neutral colors or discreet shapes, I often found myself stuck wearing a bright turquoise mask or an oddly shaped white one. When you walk around with a mask on your face and a hat on your head you may as well just write "cancer patient" on your forehead.

But, not to worry, we have all been there. I liked to think of it as a status symbol, like war paint. I told myself any stares were simply people admiring that tall, strong warrior walking by. And let's be honest, anyone staring at a cancer patient is likely thinking about how brave you are and not about how weird it is that you are wearing a mask. Quite frankly, people who may stare as you walk by in your mask are more likely scared because they are thinking about what it would be like if they were in your shoes.

I like to think of Nike's motto "Just do it" when talking about wearing masks. Just wear them because, honestly, you have to protect your insides and if it takes some wooly, turquoise thing that filters out half of the oxygen you are breathing in just to filter out all the unwanted particles in the air, then just do it! It beats an infection and more time in the hospital.

Fertility

On top of all of the treatments and preventative measures that are involved in your cancer treatment, there is fertility to worry about, and it needs your attention right away. If you are a young teenager like I was, it can be really difficult for you and your parent(s) or guardians to think ahead, about the fact that you may, in the future, want to have a family of your own. Nonetheless, my number one piece of advice is that you and your parent(s) or guardians consider and talk about this with your doctor at the very beginning of your treatment. If your doctor does not know how to address fertility during cancer treatment, ask him or her to find you someone who does, or find that second opinion yourself. In any case, it is crucial that you address this at the very start of your treatment.

So, when thinking of the bigger picture, what does this have to do with coping with cancer treatment? EVERYTHING! Making the right decision in regards to protecting your fertility means you and your support system have to be actively involved in every aspect of your treatment. Although oncologists are often amazing at what they do, they cannot be experts at everything, meaning you and your support system have to pay attention to your body too, making sure to ask the right questions. Fertile Hope is an organization that provides useful fertility-related resources and their website is included at the end of this book.

Remember, oncologists are focused on treating your cancer. It is up to you and your support system to ensure your overall health needs are addressed. If necessary, you should not hesitate to reach out to physicians in other specialties.

My own situation is an example. Guys, feel free to skip past this to the guys' fertility information in the next section.

For the girls: When I began my treatment, I was immediately put on birth control to stop my periods and the associated blood loss (anemic leukemia patients need to keep all the blood they can). However, I soon began bleeding despite being on the pill and increasing my dosage was not recommended because I had already gotten a blood clot, in part because of the pill.

Additionally, my mom was very concerned because we had been told that one of the chemotherapies I would receive had the potential to kill my eggs. Therefore, we asked for a consultation with the fertility doctor at Johns Hopkins who specialized in helping oncology patients with preserving their fertility.

My options were as follows: continue on the pill with the risk that my eggs may be affected by the chemo, have some of my eggs removed to be frozen (surgical procedure), or go on a medication called Lupron that would essentially put me into menopause and "hide" my reproductive system from the chemotherapy. We decided to go with Lupron and I received my first injection shortly after.

The common side effects of Lupron – hot flashes, mood swings, and a host of menopause symptoms – soon began. I would wake up in the middle of the night hotter than I had ever felt, and in a pool of sweat. During the day, I would get crazy mood swings and fairly frequent hot flashes. If you decide to go on Lupron, and end up with hot flashes, I found standing in front of the refrigerator with the door open was fairly useful in cooling down. Another young woman I know who has been on Lupron found eating popsicles or ice was effective to calm the hot flashes too, since those things can cool you down from the inside. Otherwise, you just have to wait for about a month or two until the worst of the symptoms subside and your body gets used to the Lupron.

For the guys: I have done some research for your side of things. It is slightly simpler for men because the most common choices for preserving fertility are sperm banking or freezing testicular tissue (Cancer.Net, 2014[3]). But, it is also a good idea for you to consult with an urologist if you want to better understand your options.

It has been six years since I completed my treatment and I can happily say that Lupron seems to have been effective for me because my reproductive system continues to function normally. While I do not know what will happen in the future – whether I am able to have kids or whether infertility becomes a problem that I do eventually face – I am so glad my parents took the time to get the help I needed. Thanks to them, I was able to make a decision that would protect my reproductive system, for the near future at least.

Radiation

While I only had two weeks of radiation during my treatment, a total of ten days, they made for ten of the most challenging days of my treatment. I was told

I would receive very small doses of radiation to my head, just enough to ensure that any leukemia cells around my brain, past the reach of the spinal chemotherapy I received, would be eradicated. It sounded great to me because I was told the dosage I would receive would result in little to no side effects, and that patients don't usually even get nauseous from it. Man, did I feel lucky for once! But, as my actual luck would have it, my two weeks of radiation were a nightmare. I became just as nauseous from the radiation as I had been during the weeklong inpatient stay during which I received the strongest chemotherapy of my entire treatment.

What was worse was that I even threw up several times, while on anti-nausea medication, which was a rare occurrence for me. On top of all that, the radiation left me feeling as if there was literally no strength in my limbs and it took immense effort to get out of my bed and get into the car each day to go for more radiation. While I realize the amount of radiation I received does not even come close to that received by so many other cancer patients, I just mention it here because it is yet another of example of how your body reacts however it wants, regardless of what doctors say "normally" happens. So, no matter what phase of treatment you are in, or what you are receiving, be prepared for the unexpected.

Overall, coping with the initial shock of treatment, learning about all of your medications and their potential risks, understanding how to manage the many side effects you may face, and protecting your fertility, are all critical for the duration of your treatment to be successful and to ensure as positive of an experience as possible.

3 LEARNING HOW TO RIDE THE ROLLER COASTER

I thought that understanding the medical aspects of cancer treatment, and learning how to get through those loops, would be the hardest part of acclimating to life as a cancer patient. Little did I know, I would still have to get to know my healthcare team, come to terms with relinquishing my dependence to parents and caregivers, and end up worrying about how my sibling was doing in the process.

Your Healthcare Team

It is crucial to develop good relationships with your healthcare team because that will help you to maintain an open and consistent dialogue with them regarding your wellbeing throughout treatment. More importantly, they can become a huge support system for you. Before you can do that, however, you need to understand who is part of your medical team and what role they play in your cancer treatment. I was treated at a large teaching hospital, so I was a bit overwhelmed at first because I had both inpatient and outpatient visits in which I saw two very different sets of staff members. I recognize that such a setup is not the case for everyone – some people may have the same doctor all the time, and just have different nurses – but I will do my best to explain a typical oncology healthcare team based on the experience I had.

First, there are the nurses. They are your go-to people and will likely become your best friends. Communicating with your nurses about any issues or concerns you have is crucial. They are your main line of support. Next, you have your doctor(s). If, like me, you are treated at a teaching hospital (in other words, a large hospital that trains doctors, such as Johns Hopkins Hospital) you will likely have both a fellow and an attending doctor.

The fellow is the doctor that will do most of your outpatient exams and discuss most of your treatment decisions with you. Your attending is the doctor you will occasionally see in clinic, or once in a while when you are an inpatient. The attending essentially oversees the work your fellow is doing, and is there in case anything serious arises that requires additional input. However, you may have two or more fellows during your treatment because of the timing of doctors' fellowships. They all, after some time, complete their fellowship, at which time they typically leave the hospital to work elsewhere as attending physicians. You also will likely have some interactions with a fellow on-call, the doctor who answers the phone after hours, for things like midnight fevers or, as in my case, spinal headaches that will not go away.

In some cases, you may also be cared for by a resident, a doctor still in training and under supervision by the fellows and attending.

With all of these different people involved in your care, it is crucial you make sure your doctor (fellow and preferably attending too) are in the loop about any problems you are having. He or she needs to know exactly what is going on, and they are not always informed by fellows on-call, etc. about what is happening with you.

In my own case, I had an awesome fellow (we can call him Dr. One) for the first year and a half of my treatment. He was there in the ER when I came in with funky blood counts. And he was there for the majority of my treatment. My favorite times with Dr. One were my outpatient visits with him. I may have been in pediatric oncology, but when I walked into the exam room, he spoke evenly to my mom, dad and me. He saw a mature thirteen year old, acutely aware of the severity of her illness, and made sure I was kept involved in all the discussions and decisions related to my care. He began all his explanations with "so..." (and this is important to note because he did, in fact, explain everything, unlike some doctors).

He taught me all about blood cells and how to interpret my blood tests. He took time to get to know me, so he learned that I was interested in going into medicine and that having cancer could be a learning experience for me, rather than just a life-threatening event. He smiled often and hugged too. He held my hand in one of my most fear-filled moments, and he celebrated with my family and me when I was in remission. When he left to go become an attending at another hospital, I was so sad he was leaving but so happy that he would be able to go and make the beginning of some other teenager's cancer journey so much easier.

Fortunately for me, the fellow who took over for him was equally wonderful (we will call her Dr. Two). She cared for me during the end of my treatment and her positivity was essential in those last few months, a time much like the end of a major marathon, during which you begin to run out of steam and are only able to keep going thanks to some cheering and positivity from the crowd. She smiled and listened intently to all my concerns. She was always good at providing understandable explanations too.

My attending situation was a little less straightforward. After the spinal headache disaster merely weeks into my treatment (and some other collective challenges), my parents grew very frustrated with the attending (we will call him Dr. A) who I was assigned to at the beginning of my treatment. They felt he was not making the best decisions for me. Therefore, they spoke with the social worker who was helping our family and requested that a different attending physician be assigned to me. That was a wonderful decision because my new attending (we will call him Dr. B) was an amazing doctor and he became a mentor to me after I finished my treatment. I actually was able to work with him on a research project during my junior year of high school, about a year after my treatment ended.

With all of that said, pediatric oncologists are certainly some of the most wonderful doctors out there. However, you and your family also have to make decisions that are in your best interest. Therefore, if you feel that the care you are receiving is not what you want it to be, or actions have been taken that make you feel compromised, do not hesitate to speak out. You may be assigned a team at the beginning of your treatment, but that does not mean you are required to keep that team.

Should you feel the need, reach out to your nurse or social worker to determine how you can make the changes you would like. Your life is quite literally in the balance and, for all you go through, you deserve compassionate and competent care. You also deserve doctors who make you feel comfortable. Your care team becomes especially important when you begin to face your first treatment challenges, which may include any or all of the medical issues I discussed in the second chapter.

A physician friend who once directed a cancer center told me that doctors, like all of us, have egos but they still want to do well by their patients. They also realize that in situations like this the doctor and patient are thrown together not by choice but by the "luck of the draw". It was Dr. A's day to take new patients when I came in, so he became my doctor just like that. My physician friend recommends that, if you do not feel your doctor is a good fit for you (for any number of reasons) a frank discussion with your doctor would be beneficial. You may want your parents to do it for you or with you. Saying something like: "Our personalities don't seem to mesh well; what do you think about trading off with one of your colleagues?" might do the trick. But, if that does not work, you should go to the top and discuss the problem with the director of the cancer center or oncology department. After all, it is your life and your treatment.

Unfortunately, I know from many other adolescent and young adult patients that compassion and competence are not guaranteed oncologist characteristics. It is very important to be aware that you have other options.

Depending on Your Parents or Other Caregivers

Normally, one's teenage and young adult years are all about gaining independence. But, when you are sick, it all changes. Learning how to depend on my parents and other caregivers was yet another major adjustment I had to make, as I learned to ride the cancer coaster. Whether you are being cared for by parents, relatives, or someone else, you may find your relationships with those people will change more than once throughout your treatment and subsequent recovery, requiring you all to adapt to those changes.

In the beginning, you will likely struggle with having to relinquish your independence to them. My saddest, most humiliating moment was when I had become so weak and sick that I could no longer bathe myself or use the bathroom on my own. As a fourteen year old, it was really hard to have to sit on a stool in the bathtub as my mom showered me. It was even harder when my mom or dad had to help me into the bathroom, pull my pants down for me, and help me pull them back up again afterward.

I found the point when you are as far away as possible from that infamous teenage sense of invincibility, and as dependent on your parents as you were the day you were born, to be one of the greatest challenges of adjusting to cancer treatment. You do not want the help but you need it. Your parents want to help you but are trying not to make you uncomfortable.

I implore you to take all the help you can get. Ask for it whenever you need it. Be strong, and do as much as possible on your own, but listen to your body and allow yourself to be helped. Initially, this new dependence may seem to strain your relationship with your parents. However, I suggest you use this change as an opportunity to strengthen your relationship with them. It was a very special moment when my mother bathed me or my dad walked with me into the bathroom.

It was so special because we were developing a bond of immeasurable trust. I would forever trust in them to be there no matter what it would require and they would forever trust me to tell them any intimate detail of my life that involved my wellbeing. I can very honestly say those difficult, yet intimate, moments with my parents made them two of my best friends.

Relationships with parents and caregivers can also become challenging if your parents or caregivers have to go back to work and cannot spend so much time with you, either in the hospital or at home. If you find yourself in this position, try not to blame or fault them for this. As you may have heard before, cancer is a family disease and an expensive one at that. Parents or guardians have to work to maintain the healthcare insurance and money to make your treatment possible. I know in my own case, my dad made this sacrifice. He worked really hard during the week, so I did not see him all that often. Fortunately, he would spend whatever free time he had on the weekends with me in the hospital, just so my mom could go home and rest. I also knew a few teens who had single parents, and I was always impressed and inspired by those teens' abilities to stay in the hospital alone and maintain as much self-sufficiency as they did.

Your Siblings

My true best friend is my little brother. He was always my baby brother, my only sibling. When I was going through treatment, I felt so bad about leaving him for days or weeks to go to the hospital. Although I did not show it and did not think about it too much, I know I felt guilty for not being there for him. I also felt so guilty that he had to help me, when I should have been there to help him through his late elementary school and early middle school years. Siblings are so important and yet so lost in the whole cancer treatment process. My mom had to be in the hospital with me almost full time and my dad still had to go to work and then find the time to visit me. That did not leave much time for my brother to get parental attention. Somehow, they still found time to go with him on camping trips with the Boy Scouts.

I wanted so much to hide my brother from the depressing hospital atmosphere, from the scary trips to the ER for fevers, from the prospect of loss. But I was powerless. Life had to go on as it did whether I was happy about it or not, whether he was ready to handle it or not. And honestly, I think I found myself more saddened and angry about the impact my treatment was having on *his* life than the impact it was having on my own.

However, now that I really think about it all, and see the amazing, mature young man he has become, I try to convince myself that maybe the whole experience was not as damaging to him as I thought. Maybe, as it was for me, cancer became a chance for him to turn adversity into opportunity. His Emergency Medical Technician (EMT) training and interest in emergency medicine have become his passion, and I am so proud of how far he has come, including becoming an Eagle Scout.

I often wonder how other patients feel, especially if, for example, his or her sibling donates his or her bone marrow or takes part in some other serious procedure in an effort to help. I can see how cancer can easily tie siblings together in an incredibly strong bond, especially when donating life saving marrow, organs, etc. But, cancer unfortunately also has the potential to break siblings apart. Fortunately, the former was the case for me, and my brother and I are very close. However, I recognize that may not always be the case, so I want to include that here as well. I know several people who struggled to maintain good relationships with their siblings during and after their cancer treatment. If you find yourself in that position, reach out to your parents, nurses, social workers, or someone else on your care team. They can facilitate ways to help bring you and your sibling(s) back together. My parents went with my brother to a psychologist during my treatment, just to provide him with an opportunity to talk to someone, in a confidential space, about how he was dealing with my treatment. It can be incredibly stressful and traumatic for siblings to go through each day unsure of whether their brother or sister will survive. This can be especially difficult for younger siblings. So, talking to a professional can sometimes be helpful for them. If nothing else, it shows your sibling he or she is still valued, despite the lack of attention he or she may be receiving because of all your treatment needs.

When just starting your treatment, I suggest this: do not worry for your siblings, do not spend your increasingly precious emotional energy on worry. Rather, act positively by letting them know you care about them. Let them know that, despite the twenty-four-seven attention you require, they are still loved and valued by you and your family. If you receive care packages or gifts, consider sharing some of them with your siblings so they can feel included. Let them know they are not forgotten. As much as we would all like things to be different, cancer is a family disease and impacts everyone involved.

Answering questions your siblings may have is a great way to keep them involved and relaxed. I do not think I did that as much as I should have. Reflecting on it now, I think that can help them be less worried about you. I know in my own case, my brother never showed he was worried about me, because he did not want me to worry about him, but his worries were expressed much more in the year or two after I finished treatment. His most notable statement was, "I felt like the only child of divorced parents." So, I know the familial separation caused by my treatment affected him, even though I failed to see it or just tried not to see it, at the time. It is also a great idea to try and have some "normal" time with your siblings. Play a game with them, take time to hang out and talk, or watch a movie together.

As a family, you can also make jokes about everything you are going through. I know this sounds crazy, but cancer jokes are very popular in my family. My dad, with his ever-present sense of humor, joked about everything from my bald head to my many medicines. The silliness we incorporated into everything I was going through always lightened the mood!

4 WHEN YOU START TO FEEL LONELY IN YOUR ROLLER COASTER CART

Two and a half years is a long time to be alone in your roller coaster cart, with only parents, siblings, and maybe a home teacher for company. Most teenagers get annoyed if they are stuck with family and away from friends for more than an hour, let alone two and a half years. The magnitude of the feeling of isolation and frustration caused by cancer treatment is immeasurable.

After I settled into the routine of my treatment, I found that isolation was, in many ways, more difficult to deal with than many of the physical challenges I experienced. In one of my journal entries from the end of my first year of treatment, I wrote, "It is like I am in this little boat all alone in the middle of this vast ocean. It is like I'm in this little rowboat, doing everything I can to survive, while everyone else my age is on this giant cruise ship right next to me, having fun and enjoying life. It is right there next to me so I can see it and hear about it, but I can never reach it." My treatment prevented me from being part of those years in which you transition from a middle school child to a high school teenager.

Many times, I wanted nothing else but to go and join that social event that I knew all my friends and classmates would be attending. Mostly I just wanted friends again. Yet, I was stuck in the hospital or at home, completely isolated from all my friends and their fun activities.

As you will unfortunately come to know, hospital rooms get very lonely, with only a parent beside you (if that) and a nurse who wanders in and out. No one else is there. You may spend weeks or months in that room, rarely leaving. Those long days cooped up in a small space can take their toll emotionally. When you finally get to go home, it is not always much better. There may be the comforts of everything you know and your family who loves you, but being stuck at home in bed or on the couch can sometimes feel like a jail cell from which you cannot escape. Sometimes you may feel hopeless and alone, knowing you still have a long road ahead of you. It can often feel like an impossible amount of time to live through. I felt like I was stuck in time, waiting for what seemed like forever, to finish my treatment. It seemed everyone around me was moving on, growing up and enjoying life.

However, I do think it is important to note that I chose to accept the isolation in order to maximize the chances of successfully surviving my treatment, and avoiding encounters with infection. This choice was not made easily, at first.

Missing School
After two months of my relapse treatment, I was on the hardest and heaviest of chemotherapies, putting me at high risk of infection because of how much it

depleted the strength of my immune system. With such a weakened immune system, and weakened body, I could not start school. I realized that, for the first time in my young life, I would not be starting school on a warm August morning, as I had done for the last eight years of my life. Worst of all, I realized that meant I would likely not see my friends for quite some time.

When all of these realizations came crashing down on me, I got mad. I was mad because learning was the one thing I was really good at – I was never an athlete, musician, or artist. I was a scholar, and I lived for the sense of accomplishment I gained from teachers' positive comments on my essays or good grades on math tests. I did not know what I would do without that, and without all of my friends. I was so angry.

When I learned I relapsed, when I suffered through the pain of my spinal headache, when I had to be put under ice to calm the fever that was trying to burn me up, when I could not get home to see my dogs, when I had to endure buckets of toxins being slowly injected into me…I could handle it. I accepted it as necessary and tried to stay positive.

This, however, was different. I realized I would be losing two and half years of school, two and a half years of friends, and two and a half years of learning. I would lose two and a half years of life that I would never get back. There was nothing fair about that and I found it difficult to see any hope in such a prospect.

That is also when my parents sat me down to talk. I will never forget the conversation either, because I know it saved me and gave me an end goal towards which I could work. My mom said, "Clarissa, you have two choices. You can go to school and risk getting an infection that could delay your treatment, and potentially be fatal. Or, you can stay home until your immune system and body recover, and keep up with your classes through a tutor. Think of it as a free opportunity for one-on-one education, to learn at your own pace and in your own way. Try and *turn this adversity into an opportunity* to learn and work towards a positive future for yourself after your treatment."

I believed that giving my body the chance to get through the chemo, without introducing infections from outside sources, would improve my chances of beating the cancer. I knew that, as hard as it would be to give up going to school, it would be the best thing for my body. So, thanks to my local home and hospital teaching program, I was able to keep up with my classes. More importantly, the opportunity to continue to learn and keep up with my studies gave me a crucial outlet. It was the only way I could remind myself there was a life to be lived after all the hardship was over. Every essay I wrote and every test I took with my home teacher, while sitting at our dining room table, was a step towards the healthy, successful future I wanted for myself.

This constant balancing act between staying on your treatment protocol while wanting a normal life makes up the most difficult challenge posed by cancer treatment. My personal belief during my own treatment was that I had one key goal – to survive the treatment. Everything else, including parties like prom or going to the mall with friends, should be secondary.

Like many teen cancer patients, I missed out on school time with friends, prom, nights out, etc. But, I accepted the short-term setback of "Missing Out" for the long-term gain of a productive and happy life. There are so many big sacrifices that you have to make while on treatment. It can be very difficult to accept them and stay positive. However, I do make the disclaimer that science and my body had the most to do with my survival. The perspective of short-term sacrifice for long-term gain is simply one I tried to maintain in order to cope and to help my mind to survive it all as well.

In the wise words of my friend Karen Shollenberger, a three-time cancer survivor, not everyone misses the same amount of school or faces the same kinds of health challenges throughout treatment, so you have to work within the bounds of your treatment to live as normal a life as possible – whatever that may mean for you. Although I missed a lot of school and activities with my peers, I did work with my doctors to plan a way for me to safely go on one fieldtrip with my classmates (while wearing my mask) and to go on a vacation to Florida with my family. So, determine what your boundaries are, including both what you are comfortable doing and what your doctors are comfortable having you do, and figure out how you can incorporate some normalcy into your treatment experience.

That being said, if you do find yourself having to make sacrifices, there *is* good to be found through those sacrifices. While I had to skip homecoming my sophomore year of high school because of the swine flu outbreak, I had the most amazing end of chemo party a few months later that brought together all my friends and family. While I missed all of eighth, ninth, and half of tenth grade because of my treatment and suppressed immune system, I was taught at home by a wonderful woman from the Howard County Home and Hospital Program, with whom I became good friends. And ultimately I graduated on schedule with my class.

Coping with the Isolation

If you want to try and get through all of the isolation with positivity, the questions then become: how do you get through the challenges involved in the short-term setback of being isolated? How do you stay in touch with your friends? How do you keep from going crazy as you walk around the inpatient unit with your IV pole for the millionth time? How do you find social and emotional support in an environment as depressing as a cancer ward?

Trying to maintain a few friendships or finding new friends is a good place to start. I know I was incredibly blessed to have had a few wonderful friends who stuck by me throughout my treatment, but I also lost plenty of friends along the way. I do not blame those friends, but I do miss the bonds we shared so long ago.

I know sometimes friends do not know how to act around you either, and others do not think to invite you because they are worried about bothering you. It is also possible that your friends do not know the first thing about cancer, and they cannot understand what you go through.

Sometimes it is necessary to explain your cancer and your treatment to your friends to help them understand. Sometimes it is also necessary to tell your friends you want them to let you know if they are getting together and that you will make the decision if you are well enough to come along, or not.

It is also important to remember that your friends are scared – for you and for themselves. Serious illness is not supposed to be a part of growing up. And it is something that we are not taught about. "What should I say to her? Should I make a joke or be serious?" Frankly, they do not know what to do so avoidance is easiest.

Although it is an incredible challenge to stay connected to friends and classmates if you are always stuck at home or in the hospital, technology these days can definitely help.

Social media can be a true lifesaver for teens and young adults going through treatment. Facebook, Twitter, Carepages, Caringbridge, online forums, and more enable you to stay connected to your friends, while also reaching out to new people. After my diagnosis, a social worker came to speak with my family and informed us about the website called CarePages. Through CarePages, my family created a blog about my treatment and posted updates on all that I was going through throughout my two and a half years of treatment. In this way, we were able to keep our family and friends all around the world regularly informed without worrying about phone calls or emails. I also received an enormous amount of support through the family and friends who visited my page and posted many caring and hopeful comments.

Because of CarePages, I also found two other teenage girls who had gone through treatment for a late relapse of leukemia, as I had. I became friends with the girls and they provided me with a great deal of advice. More importantly, they let me know that I was not alone; that my "rare" relapse did not mean my life was over.

Along with that, I had one of my friends email me or call me once in a while to give me the scoop on what was going on at school or what events were coming up so that I could stay in the loop a little.

The problem then became that I would know what was going on and be sad that I was missing it. I heard the term FOMO, or Fear Of Missing Out, used during my first semester of college. It was described as follows: that fear of missing out on key events that drives students to skip their studying in favor of the parties and fun stuff that is always happening on campus. I think FOMO takes a similar form after a cancer diagnosis. Fear of missing out by not going to school, proms, parties, and much more definitely a difficult thing to deal with during cancer treatment.

However, like prioritizing studying during college, it is crucial for you, as a cancer patient, to prioritize your recovery and wellbeing. If you decide to go to prom or a party when your counts are down, you run the risk of getting an infection that could land you right back in the hospital. If you decide to go to school for a whole week and wear yourself out completely, you could make yourself weaker rather than helping yourself maintain what strength you have left.

This, in turn, can make you more susceptible to infection. It broke my heart when I got back from my first day of ninth grade, having actually attended school, and I realized it would be far too tiring for me to go to school every day. A friend of mine, also a teen cancer survivor, was really sad about having to repeat eleventh grade because she was not able to go to school or get home tutored for a whole year. But, you can get through this challenge. I did, she did, and so have countless others.

5 THE "DOWNS"

Chemo can make you sick, isolation can make you lonely, and dependence can make you frustrated. But, when the effects of cancer treatment start to leave visible marks on your body, reminding you each time you look in the mirror of the challenges you face – that is a new kind of down.

Once you have "adapted" to the changes in your family relationships, determined how you will keep up with your classes, and developed a support system of other patients or survivors, you may feel like you have figured it out. It is also then that you find yourself in the thick of treatment. While I wish that reaching this point would mean things would get easier, emotionally it is quite the contrary. I actually found the middle of my treatment was the most emotionally challenging because I was growing tired and frustrated by how long I needed to live like an isolated invalid. I was frustrated by how long my treatment was leaving me sick and tired, a shell of what I physically used to be. The physical consequences of treatment become emotionally draining.

Hair Loss

First, we come to the topic that is often most challenging to teenage girls going through cancer treatment: losing your hair.

I will give you a little bit of a background on my hair experience. I lost my hair multiple times during my relapse treatment. When I was diagnosed with my relapse, I had very long, thick, dark hair; well past my shoulders. Before my hair began to fall out, my mom cut it short, so that the hair I did lose would be shorter.

The scariest part of that first experience with hair loss is waking up in the morning and finding more hair on your pillow than on your head. Cancer is a weird disease because you cannot see it and you cannot feel it. When you lose your hair, it is no longer possible to ignore the fact you have cancer and you are forced to confront it. Even worse, you are forced to confront the fact that, in order to live, you must let the medicines essentially destroy your body inside and out. My aunt is a nurse and described leukemia treatment as, "They will bring her as close to death as possible without killing her."

The unfortunate thing about chemo is that it comes in cycles. So, your hair can fall out and grow back and fall out again over a period of time. In my own case, I lost my hair fairly quickly. By six months into my two and a half year treatment, I was left with no hair on my head, no eyebrows, few eyelashes, and pretty much no hair anywhere else. However, the hair on my head did grow in some nice peach fuzz after I finished that most intense part of my treatment. Sadly, the first round of peach fuzz promptly decided it did not want to hang around and began leaving my head in a rather awkward fashion. For quite some time, I had some fascinating bald patches on my head!

Another thing to keep in mind is that side effects happen differently for everyone. For example, although most people lose all their hair with chemotherapy, I kept a great deal of my hair when I went through treatment as a child. Because I knew that I would likely lose all of my hair during my relapse treatment, due to the increased intensity of my chemo, I was not worried about losing it.

I was initially really uncomfortable with being bald, and definitely struggled when I was essentially hairless for the first time. I wore hats all the time, even when it was warm outside.

But, as I got further into my treatment, I began to take my hats off more often and enjoy the cooling freedom of a hairless head. I realized that it was actually quite comfortable to have no hair, especially in the summer! Rather than wearing hats all the time, I turned to big earrings to make a statement. After all, some awesome looking earrings REALLY stand out when there is no hair on your head. Also, I personally think people's faces stand out much more without hair on their head. Somehow, being bald turned into something that made me feel good about myself. It was proof that I was trying to beat the unbeatable. Now, I sometimes miss being bald, or having a buzz cut!

While I was initially uncomfortable with being bald, I was never really worried about losing my hair. On the other hand, a friend of mine, a lymphoma patient who I met in the teen room at the outpatient clinic, was terrified of losing her hair. She was not worried about scars, radiation burns, weight, etc. No, she just could not wrap her brain around the idea of losing her hair.

Now, it is important to note that she had this beautiful, waist-length blond hair, which I would be sad to lose too. She did end up losing it all, but when it grew back, I think it was even prettier because it was this warm blonde color and she had these beautiful curls. So, if the whole hair loss idea is worrying you, try to think of it as a science experiment. When else will you have the chance to shave your head, walk around with a buzz cut, or have your hair grow back in entirely different? It's like a surprise and, in the wise words of Forest Gump's mother, you never know what you're gonna get!

That being said, it is very difficult to psychologically prepare yourself to face the physical changes caused by treatment, whatever they may be. You do not really know, at the beginning, all of the physical changes you might face. You also are never sure of which changes are temporary and which ones will be permanent. I think that, no matter what physical change you face, the most difficult thing to deal with is the looks from people. Whether you are walking around the mall with no hair, sitting on the beach with your scars exposed, or sitting in a wheelchair missing a part of your leg, you feel like you stand out in that way that no one wants to stand out. I know that feeling and it is really tough to deal with at first. As teens or young adults, it is normal to want to look like everyone else our age and to like the way we look. However, with cancer that is just not possible. To prepare for those unwanted physical changes, you can make this easier for yourself by trying to relax and trying to accept that what will be will be.

You have to make a conscious decision about how you will think about yourself. If you can learn to love your scars, your bald head, your lack of eyebrows, your prosthetic…if you can learn to love your body for all that it is getting you through, you may just find yourself more content.

When you lose your hair for the first time, my advice is not to mourn the loss of it. Rather, relish the fact that you have a chance to showcase your perseverance. Do not hang your head in shame for having no hair. And realize, that one day in the not so distant future, you may actually miss that bald head of yours and all that it represented.

Weight, Scars, and Stretch Marks

Unfortunately, however, losing your hair is only one small part of a major body image struggle that can happen when your treatment drags on. For me, dealing with my body, specifically my weight, was a serious struggle.

When I relapsed, I first lost thirty pounds because I barely ate anything during the first four months of my treatment. Losing weight was not a big deal for me; I did not mind it because I thought I would get back to a healthy weight as soon as my treatment ended. When I started the Prednisone and Dexamethasone steroids, I ballooned and went right back up to my original weight, which was not really a problem either.

As I continued, I would lose a little more weight and gain a little more weight, going from steroids, to chemo, and back to steroids. The problem arose during the end of the second year of my treatment, when I was still getting lots of steroids but my chemo doses, and the frequency of my chemo treatments, decreased. This was when I gained another thirty pounds. By the end of my treatment, I had stretch marks all over the place because I had gained so much weight so quickly. I developed some pretty nice lines on my chest, stomach, legs, arms, and back from those steroids. When you go from not eating or drinking much, to eating and drinking a lot, you inevitably put on weight very quickly and skin often struggles to keep up with that growth - hence the stretch marks.

When I finished my treatment, I thought the weight and those stretch marks would start to go away, once my body began to detoxify and regain strength. Yet, I proceeded to gain another fifteen pounds in the six months following my treatment because I was eating more but still not able to exercise. This meant that from my diagnosis to six months after my treatment ended, I had gained 45 pounds. This landed me at my highest weight ever and left me with the lowest self-image I ever had.

I was okay when I had no hair anywhere on my body, I was okay when I looked as pale as a cotton sheet, and I was okay with the scars I had from my two ports, spinal taps, and various other procedures. Yet, my weight, stretch marks, and varicose veins left on my legs from countless injections really bothered me.

I just felt disgusting and old. I had the stomach of a mother of three, the thighs of an eighty year old with bad circulation, and the cheeks of a two-month-old baby. I felt so far from myself, so different from my friends and the other girls my age. They could all wear these gorgeous bikinis to the pool and flaunt their perfect teenager bodies that were toned and tanned from the sports they played or the activities they were in. I felt so gross compared to them, and it really started to depress me.

Again, it was my parents who helped me. They tried to tell me to keep in mind that my body had gotten me through hell and back; it did not matter if I looked like the other girls. I was still alive, wasn't I? I should regard my weight, my short hair, my scars, my stretch marks, and my pale skin as symbols of what I had overcome. Every time I look in the mirror and do not like how I look, I should remind myself what I have been through, what my body has been through. I have survived something that other girls my age could not even imagine.

The most important thing I needed to do was not to worry about how I looked, but to worry about being healthy. So, I started to exercise and eat healthier. That alone made me feel so good about myself because I got my body really moving again, something it had not done in almost three years. I was able to lose twenty-five pounds over the three years after my treatment ended, and achieve a much healthier weight for my height and age. I also began yoga classes that helped strengthen my muscles. Between the exercise, yoga, and a diligent moisturizer regimen I also began to notice my stretch marks became less visible.

Whether you struggle with your weight, your scars, losing your hair, or something else, remember what you are going through or what you have been through. As cancer patients and survivors, we will always be slightly different than other people our age. Try not to worry about how you look, just worry about being as healthy as possible. Accepting yourself as you are and just focusing on taking good care of your body is all that matters. In doing so, you will be able to stay positive and be proud of what you have survived. Also remember that the body is very adaptive. While it may adapt in uncomfortable ways to all of the things you go through during your treatment, you may also find it can adapt in very positive ways to a healthy lifestyle after treatment.

Depression, Anxiety, and PTSD

In handling all of these physical challenges, you may also find yourself facing some mental health challenges. As a psychology major, I have learned a great deal about depression, anxiety, and Post-Traumatic Stress Disorder (PTSD). I highlight these three because they are, I think, the most important for you to know about while going through the potentially traumatizing experiences of cancer treatment.

According to the National Cancer Institute, adolescents with cancer "…had a mean level of depressive symptoms similar to that of the general population." Essentially, that means that most patients have been shown to have great resiliency and depression is not any more common in young people with cancer than their healthy peers (National Cancer Institute, 2014[4]). However, I know from speaking with my own doctors, it is still very much a possibility. Therefore, I discuss it in an effort to make you aware of it and let you know that there are steps that can be taken to help you if you feel you are depressed.

The first step to take if you feel you may have depression would be to talk to your doctor, since he or she would be the one to get you a consultation with a mental health professional. That being said, it is up to you to stay tuned in to your mood and speak up if you feel you are struggling. Between the natural sadness and hopelessness that can come with a diagnosis of cancer and the many medications you take that alter your mood, depression is certainly something of which you should at least be aware.

Anxiety is perhaps a more likely challenge. When I was little, I think I developed some anxiety. There was a highway we had to take to get from my house to the Children's Hospital of Philadelphia, a highway that we drove countless times, and every time we would start driving on it (whether we were actually going to the hospital or not) I would begin to feel sick to my stomach. When I went through my relapse treatment, however, I thankfully did not develop that kind of anxiety. That being said, anxiety is definitely possible when you have no choice but to receive medicines and undergo procedures that cause you pain and great discomfort. Interestingly, a study screening for anxiety in adolescents with cancer showed low rates of anxiety were found from analyzing the self-reports of the patients. However, the study went on to note that, "…oncologists perceived more patient distress" (Kazak, Kersun, Mickley, 2009[5]).

So, to me, that seems to indicate we teens and young adults either do not like to admit we have a problem or we do not realize we have a problem when we do. To help you recognize these problems, it is important to know the symptoms. Symptoms of anxiety include restlessness, tension, sweating, and a host of other related symptoms that can manifest themselves in a multitude of ways (National Library of Medicine, 2014[6]).

Panic Disorder, or more commonly recognized as a panic attack, is characterized by intense feelings of dread, nausea, feeling like your heart is pounding, and several other symptoms. In either case, it is important you alert your healthcare team if you feel you are dealing with these symptoms. There are plenty of ways in which they can help you to cope, such that you can reach a point where aspects of your treatment no longer trigger anxiety and panic.

Finally, among this list of mental health challenges, we come to PTSD. I remember, back in my AP psychology class in high school, my teacher told us how soldiers are often diagnosed with PTSD or anxiety because they go through traumatic experiences in battle, fighting for their lives and the lives of others.

The soldiers are then done their tour of duty one day, and are supposed to just return home and resume normal lives the next. There is no time for them to process the trauma of their experiences and no more time to spend with the other soldiers with whom they lived and fought.

Cancer patients' experiences are so similar to those of soldiers. In fact, I think patients are soldiers, just on a different battlefield.

They fight for their lives, against their own bodies, and experience life-changing traumas. The battle can rage on for months and years. Then, one day, your treatment is just done. You are supposed to go home and start a normal life again. You have no designated time to process your traumas and you have less and less time to spend with the staff that became your second family during those months and years of treatment. Crazy, right?

It is crucial that you understand depression, anxiety, and PTSD so that you do not have to live with the impact of those disorders. Medical trauma is very real and it is important for you to get help if you think you have the symptoms. PTSD is an anxiety disorder that can cause difficulty sleeping, difficulty concentrating, repeated flashbacks of the traumatic event, and feelings of detachment. Symptoms of anxiety include excessive worry, irritability, trouble concentrating, and even nausea (Mayo Clinic, 2014[7]).

Looking on the bright side, all of these disorders can be treated and it is important that, if you feel you are experiencing any of their symptoms, you talk with your doctor or social worker so a diagnosis can be made and a treatment plan can be developed. I talk about these so you can recognize that your mental health is just as important as your physical health when going through your treatment, as well as in the months and years following your treatment.

Rumination

Aside from those more serious mental health concerns, there is another, less-official, potential psychological problem that can lead to its own challenges – "Rumination." Rumination is a word I had never heard before in my life, until I read an article about it as part of my AP psychology class, called *Lost in Thought: The Perils of Rumination*[8] by Dr. Susan Nolen-Hoeksema.

To define it simply, rumination is repetitively thinking about difficult situations and all their possible causes, consequences, and meanings without moving into problem solving. If you are wondering whether you are a ruminator, these are some questions ruminators usually think about:

"What did I do to deserve this?"

"Why do I have problems other people don't have?"

"Why can't I handle things better?"

I know I definitely did plenty of ruminating after I relapsed. While asking these questions after a serious and potentially traumatizing health experience is normal, here is the problem: According to Nolen-Hoeksema, ruminators are at a much higher risk of mental health problems, (like depression) and they have a much harder time moving past the challenges they face.

Whether you were just diagnosed, or have been going through treatment for months already, you have probably found yourself feeling like life is unfair and asking, "Why me?" You have probably found yourself ruminating. However, I want to emphasize the importance of catching yourself when you do that. You have to pull yourself out of it while you can, so that you can face the challenges and move past them.

Here is an easier way to look at it: You cannot change the situation you are in, and that admittedly sucks, *but you do have the ability to change how you deal with that situation.* In fact, the decision of how you deal with your situation is one of the few things in your treatment over which you actually have control. Take advantage of having control over that decision by deciding to adapt positively. Take time to accept the challenges you are facing, the terrible cards life dealt you. Then, stop worrying about them and think about how you can adjust your life accordingly. In a card game, terrible cards may give you a lower chance of winning, but the chance is still there. If you spend all your time ruminating about how terrible your cards are, you do not have a chance to maintain a good quality of life for yourself.

6 KEEPING YOUR HEAD UP WHEN THE RIDE BRINGS YOU DOWN

When you find yourself struggling to stay positive, tired of the disproportionate number of "downs" you have experienced relative to the "ups," try not to lose hope. There are ways to regain a positive perspective and cope with the constant feeling of life being so out of control.

Imagining Hope
When I celebrated the three-year anniversary of the end of my treatment, I thought a lot about what I went through during those two and a half years. I thought a lot about how I ever survived it all. I remember so vividly those hopeless moments, hours, days, and months of nausea, pain, and so many other forms of discomfort.

What stands out to me was the hopelessness and the intensity of it all. In such hopeless, negative, draining, horrible moments, how did I push forward? How did I convince myself to keep going, to keep taking everything that was making me feel so badly? Strangely, only now, years after I actually went through it, do I think I actually have a better understanding of how I did get through it.

I think, when there was no hope, I used my imagination to create it – I imagined hope. I dreamt about going back to school, about dancing at senior prom, about going on my first date, about graduating high school, about going to college, about becoming a doctor, about getting married. I dreamt about everything I wanted to experience in my life and it gave me hope, no matter how hopeless I felt in that moment of suffering. I imagined how incredibly wonderful all those experiences would be and how it would not be long until I reach them…I just had to keep pushing through. To really keep those ideas and dreams fresh in my mind, so that they could keep motivating me, I would often write them down in a journal or in the notes app on my phone. Keeping them as written reminders made them even more helpful and I could keep looking back at them to remind myself of the good things that were ahead of me.

Looking back on it now, having lived out more than half of those dreams I had for myself, in more wonderful ways than I could have ever imagined, I can truly say imagining hope made a difference for me.

Choosing to be a Tigger or an Eeyore
To bring to life that idea of remaining hopeful and positive, I like to use a *Winnie the Pooh* analogy. You can choose to be Tigger or you can choose to be Eeyore. In eleventh grade, my first year back at school full time, I took a computer science class for my technology education requirement. In that class we watched a movie about Carnegie Melon professor Randy Pausch that made a big impression on me. Randy Pausch is famous in the world of Computer

Science, a world I would never have taken any notice of had I not been required to take a technology class to graduate high school.

Yet, the video was incredibly inspiring. Randy Pausch passed away in 2008, after battling pancreatic cancer. The video showed his last lecture. He spoke about many things, but I will always remember his description of the difference between being a Tigger and an Eeyore. Choosing to be an Eeyore means choosing to be pessimistic, choosing to be sad, choosing to be sorry for yourself, and choosing to bring down everyone around you. Choosing to be a Tigger means choosing to be optimistic, choosing to be happy, choosing to turn this negative experience into something positive, and choosing to brighten the lives of those around you.

It was such a simple, yet profound contrast. Thinking about those words, a light bulb went on in my head. Going through cancer treatment at any age, or simply going through life, you can choose between being a positive, optimistic person or being a negative, pessimistic person. My attending oncologist once told me, "I believe very, very strongly that the degree to which a patient maintains a positive mental attitude is one of the most important factors in determining the success of the treatment." The choice is yours, but I highly recommend being a Tigger.

I almost died multiple times during my treatment, between the allergic reactions that caused me to stop breathing, the time I fainted and almost hit my head on the ground, or numerous other scary experiences. Other times I just had horribly painful issues, like the incredibly long spinal headache or when I fell down the steps because the Vincristine chemotherapy had left me with little ability to lift my feet properly.

I am sure these experiences are not nearly as difficult as the pain and discomfort that other teens and young adults with cancer have experienced, yet they were challenges to me all the same. I made a conscious decision at the beginning of my treatment that I would smile and laugh as often as possible, think positive about my future, and never feel sorry for myself. I truly believe that trying to be a Tigger, trying to be as positive and happy as possible, helped save my life. More importantly, I KNOW, that choosing to be a Tigger helped me to actually live my life as best I could in spite of my treatment.

With that idea of staying positive in mind, I want to talk about several of the major threats to being able to stay positive that you may face.

Finding Your Happy Place

The most important thing to focus on, however, is finding ways to be happy. When going through cancer treatment, I think it is absolutely necessary to have a happy place, somewhere you can go or something you can do that brings you joy and helps you get your mind off of what you are going through.

You will become familiar with the long days sitting in clinic getting chemo or sleeping through chemo on the inpatient floor. I know I wondered how I could be happy when I had so much depressing stuff going on. A hospital room gets pretty lonely, and there is usually only one parent or family member staying with you, if that. The nurses come in once in a while, but there is no one else there. You may spend weeks, sometimes even months, in the hospital. The long days of being cooped up in a small room can take their toll. Many times you may be too sick to do anything at all and cannot stay awake, so you spend your time sleeping.

When you do feel well enough to stay awake and do something, whether it be at home or in the hospital you should try doing activities that you think are fun, activities that take your mind off everything going on, activities that make you happy.

Sometimes being stuck at home is not that much better than being stuck in the hospital. Sure, there are the comforts of everything you know, but being stuck in bed or stuck at home in general can sometimes feel like a prison. Finding something that you can put your entire mind into, like arts and crafts is a really good strategy. Finding a funny movie or TV show can help too. My personal happy place was whenever I would watch my favorite TV show, *Friends*. I highly recommend that show because it makes you laugh sooooooooo hard and laughter really is the best medicine! *Friends* has ten seasons, and I watched one season during every inpatient stay. After I had seen them all, I watched the episodes over and over again and really become friends with the characters. It pulled me out of my discomfort and into this other funny, happy world. I definitely believe that finding your happy place, by doing enjoyable things that help you to feel less alone, can go a long way in boosting your mood and helping you maintain a positive attitude throughout your treatment.

Learning to Live with Purpose

Another way to help yourself focus on and maintain a positive attitude is develop a sense of purpose. When going through treatment, it is really easy to lose a sense of purpose in your life. For me, I gain a great sense of purpose and motivation from what lies ahead of me: fun with friends on summer weekends when we are not in our classes, spending my birthday weekend (July 4th) back at home with my family, and adventures to come in my fall college semester. During treatment, you lose a lot of those life-filled activities that get you excited to get up in the morning and just live. I know I found it was easy to lose that ability to look forward to the next big adventure. Even worse was that, with leukemia, the next big adventure for me was often going in for a five-day inpatient chemo trip that ended with me being utterly miserable.

So, I spent a great deal of time pondering how a cancer patient can regain some sense of purpose. How do you get excited about living a life that no one wants to live through? While I do not know if there is a definitive answer to this question, I have personally come to this conclusion: you have to temporarily refocus your purpose.

Right before I was diagnosed, my purpose in life was to do as well as I could in middle school and be a happy, healthy teen. I had a goal of being a doctor and that reinforced my sense of purpose even more, driving me to do my best in school and my extracurricular activities. But, after I was diagnosed, my days did not seem to have purpose anymore. The most I could do, because I was so exhausted from all the chemo I received, was watch TV, sleep, or read a book. Towards the beginning of my treatment, this aimlessness was a real challenge for me. I was used to a schedule, the structured life of a student. I was not used to waking up in the morning, not wanting to eat, and lying in bed all day. It was an extremely hard transition.

I was not very good at handling that transition at first and I got very frustrated by it all: missing school, missing friends, missing "normal." However, with the support from my parents, nurse, and doctor, I refocused my purpose. I made it a challenge each week to guess my blood counts and learn more about cancer from my doctor. Now I know the appropriate hemoglobin level, absolute neutrophil count (ANC), and platelet level for a person my age. I know what leukemia is and I can explain it at a cellular level to other people who ask about it.

I also tried to accomplish things once in a while, even though that was often simply painting or brushing my dogs. Painting was unquestionably my favorite though (and still is), and I will never forget how alive I felt when I went out on the back deck, during the spring of my first year of treatment, to paint. A family friend had gotten me a brand new set of paints and brushes, to go along with the canvases and easel I received from my parents for Christmas. When I set up my mini art studio on the deck, to paint and enjoy the sunshine, it was the first time I felt truly human again in over nine months. I did not realize how much I had missed being outside and being creative.

Part of my creative energy (and the only energy I had at that time) went to writing too. I wrote down a lot of what I was going through in a journal. Keeping a journal benefitted me in several ways. It helped me get out all my pent-up emotion, it helped me to recognize what I was able to accomplish in spite of my treatment, and it provided me with a way to look back on all I had been through (enabling me to gain an understanding of my experiences that I could use to help others).

My main focus, however, was studying and school work. I was determined to continue to succeed in my classes. My Math tests and English papers were the only ways in which I could remind myself I had a life to live after all the hardship was over.

Soon, I realized that I had redefined my purpose. My purpose was to accomplish little things that reminded me I had a life to live during my treatment and after I beat cancer. Whether I set out to get homework done, to watch a whole season of *Friends*, or to play with my dogs, I made sure I was consciously DOING something. Looking back on all of that, I think now that ensuring I went through each day with some sense of purpose made a big difference for me. I was able to feel somewhat capable and hopeful because of it, and I know that helped me to stay positive. Furthermore, each small thing I accomplished brought me one step closer to the end of my treatment.

So, I encourage you to set out to have a purpose each day, no matter what phase of treatment you are in. Make a to-do list, whether you are in the hospital or at home. Your purpose for the day could be to watch five episodes of your favorite TV show, get up and walk to the bathroom on your own, paint a picture of your dog, take a walk with your family, or finish a school project. No matter what it is, it matters! It matters because what you accomplish each day, however small, can remind you that there is more to your life than pills, needles, and nights in the hospital. When treatment constantly reminds you of how dependent you are, these things can remind you how CAPABLE you still are.

7 IF CANCER BREAKS THE ROLLER COASTER – GETTING OFF THE RIDE BEFORE YOU ARE READY

While treatments for cancer have come a long way since I first went through cancer treatment in 1996, sometimes science cannot reach far enough and the cancer is able to overcome the chemo. Although I do not have personal experience with this, I have known several brave teens that faced this challenge.

In their honor and in an effort to cover all of the potential challenges faced during cancer treatment, I want to talk here about what you might do if your treatment is no longer effective in fighting your cancer.

End of life care is a difficult subject to broach because it is the most emotionally charged, and it is also an area of care that is widely known for its flaws.

I read an article in the *Washington Post* (Kaminski, 2015[9]) about a primary care doctor who treated an older man for a challenging medical problem. The older man had been to many doctors, with none of them being able to help him. The primary care doctor was therefore faced with a medical mystery. Instead of sending the older man through countless more tests, the doctor decided he would reflect on words of wisdom he had learned from a palliative care doctor he knew: ask the patients what they want out of their care. It turned out the older man simply wanted to live comfortably while he could, he was not interested in prolonging his life significantly. This meant he did not actually want many more tests or doctors visits. Thanks to that primary care doctor's question, the patient finally had a chance to get what he wanted out of his care.

Many doctors do not ask such a question. If you are beginning to move towards end of life care, make sure your voice is being heard. If your doctors are not asking you what you want out of your care, then you should tell them. You may need to be forceful. Doctors do not like to "lose" and so they may even try to fool themselves. So, you may need to take the lead and force this discussion.

A study published in July of 2015 investigated the intensity of end of life care given to teens and young adults with cancer (Mack, Chen, Cannavale, Sattavapiwat, & Chao, 2015[10]).

I share their findings here because of how remarkable they are. According to the researchers, eleven percent of patients received chemotherapy within fourteen days of death. Within the last thirty days of their lives:

- Twenty-two percent of patients were admitted to the intensive care unit.
- Twenty-two percent visited the emergency department more than once.
- Sixty-two percent were hospitalized.
- Sixty-eight percent received one or more serious care measures toward the end of their lives.

But, as one pediatric oncologist noted in an article by *Forbes Magazine*, covering that new end of life care study, sometimes teens and young adults feel their quality of life is more important to them than the quantity of life they may have left (Arlotta, 2015[11]). So, when it comes time for you to make such a decision, know that it is, in fact, a choice. If you choose a better quality of life, then you have that right.

In doing some research related to this, I came across a guide, called *Voicing My Choices*. It is basically an end of life care planning guide for teens and young adults with serious illnesses. It is based on research with many, many adolescents and young adults. So, it was developed by and for people our age.

You can complete any pages that are important to you. For example, you may want to document who you want to be with you if you get very sick, where you would want to be (hospital or home), who you would like to leave important possessions to or who you would like to go through your things.

The Pediatric Oncology Branch of the National Cancer Institute and the National Institutes of Mental Health developed the guide, therefore it is a reputable resource. You complete it before you make any major healthcare changes. Should you find yourself unable to make important decisions related to your care at any point after, the book can serve as documentation of your wishes. The information about the *Voicing My Choices* guide can be found by the associated link in the resources section at the end of this book.

8 RIDING TOWARDS RECOVERY

If your cancer treatment is successful, you soon find yourself nearing the end of it. As treatment nears the end, it will suddenly get easier and less intense. You will begin feeling better, becoming more capable, taking less medication, and spending less time in the hospital. While cancer treatment is a long, drawn-out process, the end happens abruptly. From one day to the next it is all over.

The end of cancer treatment is a wonderful and exciting time, but it is also filled with its own obstacles that will challenge your ability to stay positive. Fortunately, there are ways in which you can help yourself through those obstacles, and carry your positive attitude through the completion of your treatment and beyond.

Coming to Terms with What you Went Through

If you are near the end of treatment, you have probably thought about the impending transition you will face when your treatment is over. I think a key step in care is missing during that transition. It is something called "emotional debriefing" or "decompression." Emotional debriefing means taking time to process the experiences and develop normal psychological reactions to them. Psychologists can provide this process, but I think for teenage or young adult cancer patients, it can be as simple as spending time with others who are also coming out of treatment. I found that sharing my experiences and talking about them really helped me become more comfortable with what I had been through, and it enabled me to begin to speak of it as something that no longer defined my life. Writing my blog was actually the most effective way for me to do that. You may find that blogging, emailing with other survivors, or meeting up to talk with other survivors can be effective for you. Online tools, like CaringBridge or CarePages, can help you connect with others. Alternatively organizations like the Ulman Fund for Young Adults or Teens Living With Cancer have online forums and ways to reach out to others too.

Returning to School

Going back to school is likely the first thing you do as you transition back to normal. For me, this was a momentous occasion because I had been out of school, and instead taught at home, for two and a half years. Whether or not you were out for a significantly long period of time, you may find yourself having to navigate some changes in friendships and your physical abilities. Having cancer as a teenager means that you have to miss school during some of the most formative and exciting years of your life. Whether that be middle school, high school, the transition between middle and high school, or the transition between high school and college, it can be really difficult. While friends have been busy socializing and starting new stages in their lives, many of us are thrown into a world of isolation in the hospital or at home.

While your friends spend the year(s) having fun with people their age, you spend your year(s) surrounded by the adults in the hospital who care for you, and then with your family at home. When it is time for you to return to school and to hang out with your friends, it can be incredibly difficult to get along with other teenagers.

Because I spent so many of my teenage years mostly around adults, and going through hardships my peers could never even imagine, it was really difficult for me to relate to other people my age. I found I could no longer relate to the drama, silliness, and immaturity of some middle school and/or high school students. I liked to compare my feelings to the movie *17 Again*, with Matthew Perry and Zac Efron.

I felt like (and really was) an adult stuck in a teenager's body. It can be really challenging to try to figure out how to get along with others your age after spending so much time around adults and going through something life-threatening that makes you grow up so quickly.

You may feel, many times, like you hate high school and are just waiting to move on to college, or even beyond that, to start fresh. As frustrated as you may be, it is so important to find a way to enjoy the years of school you have left, especially after missing so much. Try to accept the fact that you are going to be significantly more mature than most of your peers and that feelings of frustration and annoyance are completely normal.

The thing that helped me the most was finding other teens that had survived cancer, or another serious illness. Through similar hardships, they had become equally mature, and were often as frustrated with their peers as I was. Try to find a support group or somewhere that teens, who have or have had cancer or other serious illnesses, can get together. There was no support group in my area just for teens that have or have had cancer, so I started one with three of my friends from Camp Sunrise (the camp I go to for children and teens who have or have had cancer). I was pleasantly surprised to find out that some of those girls were also struggling with people at their high schools, and that I was not the only one. When we have issues with people and friends from our schools, we always have each other to turn to for true understanding, which is very comforting. The bright side of this challenge is that you will soon adapt to being a teenager again. Although I struggled at first, it was not long before I settled into being young again – at least for the most part.

If you are going back to school after being in treatment for a while, try thinking of your return to school as if you are going to another country and learning a new language. This can be helpful because none of your friends and classmates in school will be able to speak your language – trauma, pain, isolation, nausea, hair loss, etc. Do not expect them to understand, they simply cannot. So, take it slow and be patient.

Perhaps most importantly, *I advise you against expecting that you will get along with your old friends or that they will understand what you went through.* Your previous friends may have changed too. In your absence, their lives have moved forward and it may be just as difficult for you to understand them as it is for them to understand what you went through.

For me, this was very difficult because I really wanted to just pick up where I left off with my friends, and it did not work out well. They had changed and I could not relate to whom they had become. They were no longer people I wanted to spend time with. They had begun experimenting with partying and things that I did not want to get involved with coming out of my cancer treatment.

I sought new friends who focused on their studies like I did, and did things with them that I considered fun. Try to meet new people and make new friends, even if it means finding people in grades above or below yours, or people who do not go to your school. I first became good friends with a girl one grade above me, who I met in my math class. She had, luckily for me, been through some health challenges of her own when she was younger, so she understood at least some part of what I had gone through.

The best thing to remember is that time will make a big difference. Changes are always hard at first, but then you adapt. My first few weeks back at school were really hard, since I was learning how much everyone had changed. I found myself meeting many new people because my high school had students who came from several different middle schools.

Although being patient was difficult, it paid off in a big way. I returned to school half way through tenth grade, and despite some challenges navigating the social environment, I made it through to eleventh grade. Eleventh grade turned out wonderfully because I met some really nice girls in my English class and began sitting with them at lunch. I soon found myself becoming friends with them and becoming part of their bigger group of friends.

By the end of eleventh grade, my life had completely turned around and I had a wonderful group of friends who respected what I had been through, wanted to work as hard in school and do as well as I did, and who loved to laugh and have fun. When I first came back in tenth grade, with the realization all my old friendships would never be the same, I felt so alone. I could never have imagined how much better things would get, and that I would find friends I am still very close with to this day.

So, while the initial transition back into "reality" can be socially and emotionally draining, it is important to hope for goodness ahead and seek change when needed. In the meantime, create as much of a positive present for yourself as possible and try to enjoy the few teenage years you have left before really becoming an adult.

Saying Goodbye to Caregivers
Another challenging part of this transition back into reality is the way in

which you become caught between your new, healthy life and your old one. The separation from those nurses and doctors, who have become such an integral part of your life, presents its own emotional challenge.

At first, you will likely have regular visits to the hospital, while they watch you to ensure everything remains alright as you go off of chemotherapy entirely. Yet, you will be integrating into your school and healthy life more and more. The day you celebrate receiving your last chemotherapy treatment is unquestionably one of the greatest days of your life. But, for me, I think it was also a little bit of a sad day.

Looking at the end-of-chemo cake my healthcare team had gotten me, reading all of the messages they wrote to me on my "You Did It" t-shirt, and looking around at them singing "Happy End of Chemo to You," gave me this sinking feeling. Behind all of the happiness, I realized that I might never see some of them again. Those people who smiled and sang around me had saved my life. They became my best friends and second family. I had clung to their smiles and words of care for so long, I did not know what I would do without them.

As I progressed farther and farther from treatment, however, I found I disconnected more easily than I expected. All too soon my worry changed from worrying about not seeing them anymore to worrying about forgetting them. To me, forgetting them meant I would be forgetting what that time in my life meant to me – that was scary too.

This worry became even more prevalent to me one night at the cancer camp I attend every summer. It was August of my second year post-treatment. I was a Counselor In Training, and I was enjoying the campfire with my campers. As I walked over to get a water bottle for one of my campers, I ran into my attending oncologist, and got so excited. Standing next to him was a nurse and, as I looked to her, he asked, "Remember her?!" with a smile on his face.

My heart sank and mind raced as I failed to recall her name, despite how familiar her face seemed. When she reminded me of her name, I hated myself because I remembered she was one of my favorite inpatient nurses. She had been there with me during some of the hardest moments of my life and I did not even remember her name. I felt so guilty and so sad. It made me realize there would probably come a day when much of what I went through would be hard to remember.

While that should really be a good thing, for me it was incredibly sad because I regard my journey through cancer treatment as the most defining experience of my entire life and a huge part of me never wants to forget it.

As with everything else, I found I adapted. I still miss my doctors and nurses dearly, and although I will not likely remember all of their names I will write enough down in my journals and the pages of this book to remind me of what they did for me.

However, some of you may find you want to get as far away as possible from all things cancer, which is also perfectly normal (basically you cannot go wrong either way).

Losing Friends and Fellow Patients to Cancer

With all that said, there were many parts of my transition back into "reality" to which it was not so easy to adapt. I must admit, as much as I am a proponent of thinking positively, there are certain events both during and after my treatment that have put my positive attitude to the test. One of those events is learning another young life has been lost to cancer. The first time this happened to me was the hardest; it was devastating.

I first experienced the loss of a fellow cancer patient when the teenage boy who had been diagnosed with the same ten-year-later relapse of leukemia, around the same time as I was, lost his battle.

For the first time in my entire treatment, it dawned on me that I could have been the one who did not make it. I guess everything had gone relatively well throughout it all, such that I never had to think much about what would happen if my treatment did not work.

Strangely enough, I never thought twice about dying from my cancer. To me, it was never an option or a possibility (even though it really was). I was given a forty percent chance of survival (leaving me with a sixty percent chance of not surviving) at my diagnosis, but I never thought that such a statistic would hold true.

So, I could not comprehend why that boy had to be given the worse half of those odds. I felt guilty because I had taken the good part of our odds. I never really told anyone how I felt about that; I just did not think they would understand because not many cancer patients are diagnosed with a rare cancer at the same time as someone else, get to know that person, and then go on to survive while the other person does not. It is kind of like the soldier who survives when his buddies die or the car accident victim who loses all others in the car. In all cases, there is guilt.

After I finished my treatment, and even as I write these pages, I learn that some survivors I know have relapsed for the second or third time. Some have recently had bone marrow transplants that have left them fighting massive complications. Another young person lost her battle and passed away peacefully only a few months ago. Many of these teens are or were my friends. I cannot help but wonder why.

I get angry, I cry, I pray, I hope, I hurt. While my first confrontation with mortality left me feeling guilty and frustrated, these others leave me with yet another host of feelings: heartbreak, terror, and inspiration all interwoven together.

The news was heartbreaking because yet another life is lost, a young life that was filled with so many hopes and dreams. The girl that passed away did not ask for this to happen to her and it just seems so unfair. It makes me cry thinking of how she will never get to live out her life and reach all of her dreams.

Despite the unfairness of it all and the sadness you may feel with such news of loss, as survivors we are again left with a choice to make. Do we let ourselves drown in all that loss, or do we try to make the most of what we have and choose to be inspired by the lives that were lost? I choose the inspiration route. Once I had finished my treatment, I was at cancer camp for my first summer as a Counselor In Training and was told that one boy who would be coming was nearing the end of his battle and that it would likely be his last year at camp.

Apparently that boy had two wishes to fulfill before he died: to complete ninth grade and to go to one more week of Camp Sunrise. He fought so hard that he made it out of the hospital and was able to finish ninth grade. Then, he fought harder to make it to camp for the whole week, even if it meant going home each night and coming back each morning or afternoon. He finished the week at camp with everyone else. Just two weeks later, he died peacefully.

He completed both his goals. To me, and I believe to everyone that knows him, he will always be a shining example of strength, perseverance, and motivation. As cancer patients and survivors, there is so much we can learn from the loss of such a life. First, it should remind us of where we have come from, so that we may fight equally as hard to set and to reach our goals as that boy did. Secondly, if we can live full, positive, and useful lives, maybe those young lives were not taken in vain – maybe we can help bring purpose to their existence.

After all the times my heart has sunk and my eyes have welled with tears, after all of the helplessness and fear I have felt, it took me a while to feel like I was once again on solid ground. Why? Well, I think it is because I see cancer treatment from the sidelines for the first time.

I see the way some amazing young people are handling all of the incredible unfairness that they have been dealt. I see the way their families, friends, and communities rally together to support them. I see the way they smile and exceed the expectations of their doctors. I see the way they persevere. I see the way they handle tragedy with incredible grace and courage.

It is from their examples that survivors must learn. As survivors, we are blessed with having lived through something that could have killed us. That being said, we are all the more prone to emotional reactions towards hearing that others have to face what we know all too well, or that others have not made it through the same disease we fought.

Therefore, as much as we have learned from our own experiences, we must also learn from the experiences of others. We must remember not to spend too much time being sad, asking why, getting mad, or feeling hurt. We must allow ourselves a short time to feel those feelings and then move on.

If we can be like Tigger, we will help ourselves so much and have the potential to help others as well. More importantly, we must remember that fight instinct that kicked in right after being diagnosed. We have to remember that instinct that told us we had no choice but to persevere, however unfair life may seem.

9 STEPPING OFF OF THE ROLLER COASTER, INTO SURVIVORSHIP

The fresh start you get when finishing cancer treatment can be exhilarating. But, for me, the beginning of "normal" life tested me. I thought I had learned patience, open-mindedness, and how to maintain peace of mind. I thought cancer had already taught me enough important life lessons. I was so wrong about that though.

I think I had wanted so much to maintain control over my life, that when I finally had control again, I became anxious, impatient, and closed-minded about many things. That was not so good for my emotional wellbeing. I am still struggling to let go of things, and thankfully college has begun to help me let go of what I cannot control, learn to let life happen with patience, and be open to new opportunities. There is a saying I like to think of that says:

"Grant me the Serenity to accept the things I cannot change,
the Courage to change the things I can, and
the Wisdom to know the difference."

While I am still fighting against anxiety (something I think seems to be a natural product of overcoming one life-threatening event and not ever wanting to encounter another one), I feel like I am finally inching closer to living out that serenity, courage, and wisdom for which I prayed.

To save you from falling into the same traps as I did, I advise you to be patient, calm, and open-minded as you start life again. Life will always throw you curveballs and you can lose yourself in the uncertainty of that, as I did for a time, or make the best of each day and try to have the best quality of life possible.

This is especially crucial as you transition from patient to long-term survivor.

The Beginning of Survivorship

When I first finished my treatment, the aspect of survivorship that I began to most appreciate was regaining my independence. I often think back to the times when things were not so normal and I had absolutely no independence at all. I went from being incapable of bathing myself to getting my drivers license and applying to colleges within a matter of two years. Just as the change to dependence after your diagnosis presented a challenge to the relationship you have with your family members, the same goes for this transition back to being independent.

I still laugh at my mom when, almost six years after finishing my treatment, she goes to stand in front of me on escalators or tells me to be careful walking down steps. When I had just finished my treatment, I would get really annoyed because I knew I was capable again and could not understand why she would not just leave me alone and let me take care of myself. It was not until I got really mad at her one day, for making a comment about it being important for me to be careful on the stairs, that I took a minute to understand her side of it.

I failed to recognize that she and my dad had spent so long doing so much for me, and watching me suffer so much, that they would take much longer than I would to regain a sense of safety regarding my capabilities. Mom was the one who caught me when I fainted because my red blood cell count was too low, dad walked me to the bathroom when I could not do it myself, mom bathed me when I could not do it myself, dad had to work to make me laugh when everything else was making me feel awful, and mom held my hand walking down the steps when Vincristine left me with little control over my feet.

I had zipped so quickly into my "normalness" I had completely forgotten that my mom and dad might not find it so easy to bounce back. So, when going through this post-treatment transition, keep in mind your parents and family members are transitioning too. You will not all transition at the same pace and it will affect you and your family members differently. That being said, when you are capable once again, but still like to use your little brother to go upstairs and get things for you, or do the dishes because you are "still too tired," do not be surprised if your parents (and little brother for that matter!) begin to call you out on it. Becoming independent again means acting like the capable young person you are becoming, and pulling your weight in the family again (I learned that one the hard way).

Talking About Your Cancer

When transitioning into survivorship, I think there is a frequently overlooked issue out there among teens and young adults with cancer: the whole do I tell people about "it" or not. By "it" I mean the fact that you had cancer. Some people never want to say anything about it. As for me, I really struggled, and continue to struggle, with the fact that no one knows what I have been through. I just did not know whether to talk about it or not because, when I walk down the street, start at a new school, or join a new activity, no one knows about my past.

But, I have also found that my memories of what I went through are like all these balloons in my mind: they float up at random times and no matter how much I try to push them back down into the background, something always triggers them to float back up. If we are talking about the fact that the American Red Cross is running a blood drive at Duke and my friends are debating whether to donate blood, all I can think is how many bags of platelets and red blood cells I got and how much I want them to donate blood so that they can save lives like mine, lives that would otherwise not have lasted if it were not for people who donate. When the student health clinic comes to give free flu shots and everyone at my dinner table starts talking about how they hate needles, all I can think of is the hundreds of needles that have pierced my skin. The list goes on and on.

I thought it would be weird, and I thought people would think of me differently, if I just brought up random things about my treatment related to the conversation. I would have trouble in trying to describe my high school experience or the activities I did (which is basically all you talk about the first weeks of college) without bringing up my experiences with cancer. Basically, I was finding it hard to talk about myself if I did not also talk about my cancer. I thought I could not talk about my experiences and still be able to start over without being branded as "that girl who had cancer."

When I started college, I was so unsure of what I wanted to do about this big secret of mine: the fact that I survived cancer twice. I had no idea if I could or should talk about it with people. My family was curious as to what I wanted to do about it too. Do I tell people if it comes up in a conversation and deal with the "ooohhhhss" and "ahhhs" and questions, deal with the fact that people can never understand even if I tell them? Or do I keep it to myself and take this as an opportunity to start over? I thought it was an either/or situation…but that could not have been farther from the truth.

I realized that my experiences with cancer shaped me and became an important part of my past. Along with that came the realization that I was proud of what I have been through and what I have been able to do with my life since then. I came to understand that if I want to tell people about what I've been through because it is important to whatever else I am talking about, then I should be proud to do so and have the confidence to share my story.

I decided, if the people I talked to would look at me differently because of it, then I needed to find better people. So, I started talking to people about it, sharing with them these pieces of me, and I found it was so rewarding in so many ways. First of all, I felt relief simply by saying something about my treatment. Second, I think it allowed people to better understand me, which has helped deepen my friendships.

The best thing was that the people with whom I have talked to about it, even just in casual conversation, know that about me and do not make a big deal about it like I thought they would. More importantly, I have actually brought it up in multiple conversations with new people. They responded by telling me about someone they knew who has or had cancer and how inspirational it was to know I was able to get through it and get to where I am today.

I think it can be difficult for young people to talk about having or surviving cancer because it is such a taboo subject still. People always associate it with death and unimaginable things (which is unfortunately part of it sometimes), so people can react to it in various ways. But, more and more people are surviving cancer as treatments continue to improve. I think it is very important for survivors to have confidence in themselves and their stories because it is talking about what you have been through that helps you feel like you are letting go of this big secret.

I had been holding my secret in for a while now, and it feels so good to really acknowledge that part of my life and who I am. The best part about talking about your experience with cancer is that you may unknowingly provide a story of hope for someone who has cancer or who knows someone else with cancer.

Fear of Relapse

Talking about your experience with cancer can often be troublesome though, because it means you have to think about what you went through. For me, that can sometimes make me worry about if I will ever have to go through it again. Making a fresh start after treatment ends is often hampered by the fear of relapse. And so we come to the crucial topic of how to deal with that fear. How do you live in spite of the fact you will never know if or when your cancer could or would come back? For me, this is especially challenging because it has already come back once in my life, and it did so a decade after I had it the first time, so I do not know if I will ever truly feel safe from it.

While I do think that cancer can be as much of a blessing as a curse, because it unites people, refocuses people on what is important, and provides motivation to persevere, I fight every single day against the fear of it coming back again. All it takes to scare me is a fever, a bruise, or feeling tired. This is, of course, made even worse by the fact I happened to relapse ten years after my first diagnosis, which has a less than one percent chance of happening….but it did. Because of this, I can never figure out whether the odds will be in my favor.

I like to relate the whole cancer relapse issue to Harry Potter. One snowy weekend last winter, my family watched all eight Harry Potter movies, just because we had never really seen them sequentially and we thought it would be fun! So, I will get a little nerdy here and note that you can relate cancer to Voldemort. In my case, I had beat "him" over a decade ago and never anticipated he would threaten my life ever again.

However, little did I know, he must have been gaining power all those years because he returned very suddenly, and attacked without hesitation or mercy. Much like Harry in the last Harry Potter movie, I had the choice to fight him myself or cause all of my family and friends to suffer unimaginably. Since the clear choice was to fight, that was precisely what I did.

Yet, despite the fact I am almost a six-year relapse survivor, I sometimes find myself worrying if he will ever return again. If I see bruises on my legs, or I feel unusually tired, or I get dizzy when I stand up, that anxiety creeps up on me. While that anxiety used to be more of a challenge for me, I have come to learn not to dwell on it.

Before worrying unnecessarily, I first of all recommend you get the facts from your doctor. While I am not a huge fan of statistics (simply because I had less than a one percent chance of relapse but it happened anyway), it might make you feel better to know the statistics for your cancer (if there are any).

More importantly, though, you have to stay positive – with or without those statistics. I like to think of a quote from baseball player Mickey Rivers to describe why positivity and staying as worry-free as possible are essential:

"Don't worry about things that you have no control over,
because you have no control over them.
Don't worry about things that you have control over,
because you have control over them."

You have no control over whether or not you relapse, so do not waste your time worrying about it. You have complete control over your attitude and outlook on life, so concentrate on making those as positive as possible. However, I definitely acknowledge that this is easier said than done. Therefore, I highly recommend that you get extra help if you think you need it! There are many resources out there to help you deal with the fear and anxiety caused by the uncertainty of relapse, so do not hesitate to get help before you lose yourself in the fear (which has happened to plenty of people before, so you would not be alone in that). My dad told me about a saying from Chinese philosopher Lao Tzu that I think provides the best perspective:

"If you are depressed you are living in the past.
If you are anxious you are living in the future.
If you are at peace you are living in the present."

10 LONG-TERM HEALTH

I participate in an email thread with other cancer survivors through a scholarship program, run by a national cancer support organization. One of the most recent email exchanges was about something very important: an alarming number of young adult survivors get lost in transition after treatment. Yet, the transition into follow-up care is so important for your mental and physical wellbeing after treatment. I feel lucky to have had great guidance in terms of late effects because I am part of the survivorship follow-up program at Johns Hopkins. I see my doctor there once a year. She follows my academic performance, physical abilities, and more.

Academic Challenges

This was immensely helpful during my first semester of freshman year, when I found myself really struggling to finish my exams within the given time. I had never had any trouble academically, so I had no idea I could eventually have issues from the chemo and radiation I received. However, when I went to my survivorship appointment that winter, my doctor told me that delayed processing ability, as seen in having trouble completing tests in the given time, is quite common for survivors of many pediatric cancers. In fact, a variety of cognitive issues are common for young people in the years following the completion of their cancer treatment.

Typically, issues arise in either the ability to process information or with executive functioning skills (i.e. planning ahead and time management). She said it definitely seemed that I was having trouble processing information, so she helped me get in touch with Duke's Office of Student Disabilities. Coming to Duke, I never even knew such a place existed, so it was very helpful to learn about that. Through their help, I was able to get an accommodation for extra time on tests, and it has been an immense help. For example, my calculus grade improved by a whole letter grade by simply getting more time to take my tests. For those of you who, like me, find yourself in a bit of a chemo brain fog once in a while, this is a really useful accommodation.

Physical Health Challenges

The doctors working in these survivorship programs are also very familiar with all the current survivorship research. This was useful to me when I was struggling to get back to a healthy weight after gaining a great deal of weight from being on high-dose steroids during my treatment. My survivorship doctor was able to tell me about recent research that was showing leukemia survivors can often have decreased metabolic function, so they may have a harder time maintaining a healthy weight. Through this information, I learned to be more careful of my diet in order to maintain a comfortable, healthy weight. Any issues like this that you find important can be better understood through such follow-up care.

Accessibility and Usefulness of Participation in Follow-up Care

For all teenage and young adult survivors, I strongly recommend becoming part of a survivorship program and making time for such follow-up visits. I have found it so useful and encouraging, even just to know, year after year, that I have not experienced many of the issues common for survivors of my cancer.

Many major hospitals have long-term follow up services in their oncology clinics. You can also find some useful information about follow-up care after cancer on the National Institute of Health (NIH) website, which you can find in the resources at the end of this book.

The Emotional Impact of Survivorship Health Problems

The other challenge that underlies all of these potential physical difficulties after treatment is the emotion factor. When I was struggling academically during freshman year in college, I was so confused as to why it was happening. I did not understand why I had trouble thinking straight sometimes. I was annoyed by the fact that on science and math tests I would often need to read the question a bunch of times before my brain would register what the question actually meant. More importantly, I was terrified about what it could mean.

My entire identity has been built around my academic achievements. Because my cancer treatment as a toddler had, shall we say, not been an enabling force in development of athletic ability, I had to do other things. Music ended up not being my favorite activity either. But, I loved school. So, I spent my life cultivating my academic talents. I excelled in high school and made it to my dream university. I was so proud of myself for getting there, for proving to myself I was really good at something. When I began to struggle, I was so scared by the possibility that I could lose that academic ability of which I was so proud. If I lost that, what would I be left with? That fear definitely began to stress me out.

What was worse was that I knew extra time on tests would again make me "different" because you end up taking your exams in a separate room, such that you can work in peace and the timing does not conflict with the work of other students. While that is a great system, it is difficult to get used to when you are a cancer survivor and just want to feel "normal." Somehow, I was yet again forced to get through situations that filled me with sadness, anger, and fear.

But, I am incredibly grateful for my annual visit with my survivorship doctor that happened over the winter of my freshman year. It is thanks to her that I was able to learn that I was, in fact, experiencing a challenge quite "normal" for young cancer survivors. I was normal when looking at the group to which I will forever belong: the survivors. And understanding what is "normal" for you, as a survivor, is the most important reason for visiting a survivorship specialist regularly. You can trust me when I say that denying physical or cognitive challenges you may be experiencing will probably lead you to some bad outcomes.

It has also helped me to realize that these challenges are, in some ways, a good thing because they have led me in so many different directions. My academic struggles in college led me to move away from my lifelong dream of becoming a doctor. However, they also enabled me to open my mind to other opportunities, such that I could realize my true passion is in psychology. Becoming a clinical psychologist for young people with serious illnesses is now my goal. I never would have been able to figure that out, had I not struggled so much to get through my premed classes.

"Life is What Happens When Your Plans Fall Apart"

I like to quote one of my psychology professors who shared with my class something he had heard from his neighbor: "Life is what happens when your plans fall apart."

It is a simple statement, but one that provides me clarity in my moments of fear and doubt. It helped me to remind myself that recognizing there is a problem simply leads to getting help to fix it. A challenge is not necessarily the end of anything. In fact, challenges can often lead you to new and interesting beginnings. Furthermore, I have recognized that it is okay to ask for help. There is no shame in admitting a struggle. I did not realize how fiercely independent and averse to assistance I had become since finishing my treatment. I had no idea that being so dependent for so long would make me so resistant to anything involving getting help. But, thinking about it now, that is definitely what happened.

When I found myself struggling with time management during my junior year, I knew I needed help and, learning from my struggle freshman year, I recognized that I could not get through it on my own. So, in addition to continuing to request extra time on exams through my school's disability office, I also began meeting with a learning specialist at Duke's Academic Resource Center.

It was the best decision because I walked out of that meeting with hope. I did not feel alone and I no longer felt defeated. I no longer felt that I had completely lost my one shining talent, and I knew that the woman I met with was going to do her best to help me in all aspects of my academic life. From time management skills to study techniques, she worked with me to help me improve. The skills that were most helpful to me were related to time management. She printed out a semester calendar for me and we wrote all my major exams, projects, essays, and such into the calendar so I could visualize when my biggest assignments were due. Then, she printed out a weeklong calendar in which I spaced out all of my homework for the week based on what I thought I could get done. Doing all this planning one day each week helped me be less anxious about getting it all done during the week, because I knew we had spent time fitting it all together such that I could make it work. Also, I found it so helpful to hear about her experiences with other students so that I could recognize I was not the only one seeking help.

In understanding what is "normal" for you as a survivor, the three most important things to remember are:

1. Recognize when something does not feel right and, instead of getting scared, get information.
2. Talk to a survivorship specialist about it or look it up on your own, using a reputable source, so you can understand what you are dealing with.
3. Recognize it is okay to be a little dependent on someone for help – time management assistance or meetings at the office of student disabilities do not revert you back to patient status!

Basically, I have a choice. I can sit here and be bitter about the late effects from chemo and radiation, or I can accept it and do my best with what I have. I can choose to think like Tigger or I can choose to think like Eeyore.

When confronted with late effects, or any health challenges that threaten your life plans, recognize it is part of this life you have been given. Remember too that you have been given a second chance at life, and find out how you can work through the challenges you face. Whether it be seeking academic assistance or admitting your physical capabilities may never be the same and seeking support for that, do not hesitate to ask for help. You may find regular checkups with a mental health care provider would be useful for you so that you do not have to emotionally "catch up" years after your treatment, as I think I may have done. I also encourage you to maintain contact with other survivors, or some kind of support community, that gives you the opportunity to recognize and appreciate the significant life experience that is living through cancer.

There is no shame seeking support, and no one can know you are struggling unless you say something. While you may be free of your illness, your body and mind will likely be forever affected by it. But, most important of all, *remember you are not the only one.*

11 PUTTING IT ALL TOGETHER

In my quest to find resources for young people going through cancer, I got tired of looking for books directed at actual young people with cancer because, well, I just did not find many and what I did find missed the very content for which I was searching.

So, I decided to check out the academic section of my local bookstore to see what psychology-related content I could find. Surprisingly, there was actually a psychology section. While half of it was filled with some very creatively titled self-help books, it seemed the other half was filled with books on serious mental illness.

Just as I began to wonder if I would find anything useful, in the middle of the shelf I found an interesting book by Mihaly Csikszentmihalyi titled *Flow: The Psychology of Optimal Experience*[12]. While the "optimal experience" part sounded a little strange, I thought I would check it out. I was sold by the following quote from the first chapter:

> "What I discovered was that happiness is not something that happens. It is not the result of good fortune or random chance. It is not something money can buy or power command. It does not depend on outside events, but, rather, how we interpret them. Happiness, in fact, is a condition that must be prepared for, cultivated, and defended privately by each person. People who learn to control inner experience will be able to determine the quality of their lives, which is as close as any of us can come to being happy."

While I do not totally agree with everything he says, because I think it is hard to completely control one's inner experience, I do believe he hits the nail on the head in saying happiness depends on how we interpret what happens to us and how we prepare for it, cultivate it, and defend it. Csikszentmihlyi writes that being able to do all of that enables you to have what he calls "optimal experience."

Let's be real though…how much "optimal experience" is going on in oncology clinics? That was my question…until I thought about it, and realized…how do the little kids who go through something as awful as cancer treatment still manage to wander around the playroom smiling and playing as if they noticed no difference between that playroom and any other playing space? Their childhood was happy, and then something came and threatened it. But, as kids, they are naturally happy and cultivate happiness, sharing it with those around them. So, when their happiness was at risk, they defended it by playing, just playing, by finding the toys in the midst of IV poles, baldness, and masks.

It got me wondering if they might just have this whole thing figured out. I wonder if we can prepare to be happy, to cultivate happiness, and to defend our happiness when it is threatened, by doing what those little kids in the playroom do.

Even if you are not looking to play with Legos or dolls anytime soon, you could find a thought-provoking book or do something else that helps you cultivate your happiness. Do something you enjoy at least once a week. It makes such a difference. Most importantly, however, think about your perspective, how you interpret the things going on in your life.

Here are a few examples of times when something exceptionally frustrating, painful, or scary happened. I distinctly remember something positive happening in the midst of or after these events, and I chose to interpret the challenging experiences simply as prequels to some of the most amazing moments of my life.

Bad	Good
I suffered through a painful spinal headache for twenty-eight days.	At the end of the twenty-eight days, I found out I was in remission.
The H1N1 Flu outbreak meant I would not be allowed to go to my tenth grade homecoming dance.	Shortly after, I returned to high school after having been absent for two years.
I wore a bathing suit around my peers for the first time, revealing the stretch marks on my arms and legs from the steroids, as well as the nice big scars from my two ports.	No one noticed or cared, and I had the most amazing time at the pool with all of my friends.
I received a 40% on several of my organic chemistry tests, threatening my medical school dreams.	My friends happened to have been struggling with something too and we all decided we would do something fun together to get over the bummer of the bad grades.
I did not get accepted to a really awesome summer internship in a Neonatal Intensive Care Unit (which would have been the greatest premed opportunity).	I ended up back at Duke doing a summer research practicum in the lab of one of my psychology professors, which was an incredible learning experience that guided me towards choosing to become a clinical psychologist.

Everyone's experiences in life are different. More importantly, no one faces challenges the same way. But, no matter what challenges you have faced, you may benefit by changing the way you think about those challenges.

First, think of challenges as "all relative". Einstein's theory of relativity pertained to physics and the movement of objects in space and time. My theory of relativity is the theory of the relativity of suffering, and it pertains to the reality of facing challenges over time. Basically, the underlying point is that looking at suffering and challenges as all relative to your current level of experience can help to recognize the positives in whatever challenge you are facing. For me, this perspective continues to help me to see the good in whatever bad I may face.

When you think about your experiences, you can interpret them however you want. I was diagnosed with and survived cancer twice. For me, that was the greatest challenge of my life thus far, and I compare all my other challenges to it. In doing so, I see that there are few other challenges in my life as difficult as that was. I thereby feel empowered and able to overcome so much more because I understand any challenges I face now cannot be as bad as two and a half years of cancer treatment.

Secondly, I also chose to learn from the experiences I had throughout my cancer treatment. Turning it all into one big learning experience has taught me so much about myself, but it simultaneously has enabled me to help others who are trying to overcome serious illness.

I encourage you to take some time to find out the best way to make your life experiences optimal experiences :-) Cancer, and any major challenge really, can seem like a barrier to what you are trying to achieve. However, such obstacles can also serve as motivators and reminders to live fully. The way you perceive your challenges is your choice, so choose wisely.

RESOURCES

You can find teenage and young adult cancer resources and read my blog at www.teen-cancer.com. I have also compiled the following list of several useful organizations and websites.

- *American Childhood Cancer Organization:* http://www.acco.org/

- *CancerCare:* http://www.cancercare.org/

- *Children's Hospital of Philadelphia Center for Pediatric Traumatic Stress:* http://www.chop.edu/centers-programs/center-pediatric-traumatic-stress

- *Johns Hopkins Pediatric Oncology Patient Stories:* http://www.hopkinsmedicine.org/kimmel_cancer_center/centers/pediatric_oncology/patient_stories/

- *Fertile Hope:* http://www.fertilehope.org

- *Group Loop:* http://www.grouploop.org/

- *Moving Forward Cancer Series:* https://www.youtube.com/watch?v=F7kHCaPAsF4&list=PLD3FB007EC0755947

- *National Cancer Institute Resources for Adolescents and Young Adults:* http://www.cancer.gov/cancertopics/aya/resources

- *National Cancer Institute Information about AYA Cancer:* http://www.cancer.gov/types/aya

- *National Children's Cancer Society:* https://www.thenccs.org/

- *National Institutes of Health* Follow-up Care Information: http://www.cancer.gov/cancertopics/factsheet/Therapy/followup

- *Ped-Onc Resource Center:* http://www.ped-onc.org/treatment/teencancercare.html

- *Planet Cancer:* http://myplanet.planetcancer.org/

- *Stupid Cancer:* http://stupidcancer.org/

- *Teenage Cancer Trust:* https://www.teenagecancertrust.org/

- *Teen Cancer America:* http://teencanceramerica.org/

- *Teens Living with Cancer:* http://www.teenslivingwithcancer.org/

- *Ulman Cancer Fund for Young Adults:* http://ulmanfund.org/

- *Voicing My Choices:* http://www.agingwithdignity.org/voicing-my-choices.php

- *2bME:* http://lookgoodfeelbetter.org/2bMe/2bMe.html

REFERENCES

[1] Cancer Research UK. (2008). *Teens' and young adults' cancer incidence in Europe and worldwide.* Retrieved from http://www.cancerresearchuk.org/health-professional/cancer-statistics/teenagers-and-young-adults-cancers

[2] Bowen, M. & Godfrey, W. (Producers). Boone, J. (Director). 2014, June 6. *The Fault in Our Stars* (Motion Picture). United States of America: 20th Century Fox.

[3] Cancer.Net. (2014). Fertility concerns and preservation for men. *Sexual and Reproductive Health.* Retrieved from http://www.cancer.net/navigating-cancer-care/dating-sex-and-reproduction/fertility-concerns-and-preservation-men

[4] National Cancer Institute. (2014). Depression- for health professionals. *Feelings and Cancer.* Retrieved from http://www.cancer.gov/cancertopics/pdq/supportivecare/depression/HealthProfessional/page7

[5] Kazak, A., Kersun, L., Mickley, M., & Rourke, M. (2009). Screening for depression and anxiety in adolescents with cancer. *Journal of Pediatric Hematology/Oncology, 31*(11), 835-839. Retrieved from http://www.ncbi.nlm.nih.gov/pubmed/19829153

[6] National Library of Medicine. Anxiety. *MedlinePlus.* Retrieved from http://www.nlm.nih.gov/medlineplus/anxiety.html

[7] Mayo Clinic. Post-traumatic stress disorder (PTSD). *Diseases and Conditions.* Retrieved from http://www.mayoclinic.org/diseases-conditions/post-traumatic-stress-disorder/basics/symptoms/con-20022540

[8] Nolen-Hoeksema, S. (n.d.). *Lost in thought: The perils of rumination.*

[9] Kaminski, M. (2015). A doctor discovers an important question patients should be asked. *The Washington Post.* Retrieved from http://www.washingtonpost.com/national/health-science/how-i-discovered-an-important-question-a-doctor-should-ask-a-patient/2015/03/09/ca350634-bb9c-11e4-bdfa-b8e8f594e6ee_story.html

[10] Mack JW, Chen LH, Cannavale K, Sattayapiwat O, Cooper RM, Chao CR. (July 2015). End-of-Life Care Intensity Among Adolescent and Young Adult Patients With Cancer in Kaiser Permanente Southern California. *JAMA Oncology, 1*(5), 592-600. Retrieved from http://oncology.jamanetwork.com/article.aspx?articleid=2383144

[11] Arlotta, C.J. (2015). How do young adult cancer patients want to spend their final days? *Forbes.* Retrieved from http://www.forbes.com/sites/cjarlotta/2015/07/10/how-do-young-adult-cancer-patients-want-to-spend-their-final-days/

[12] Csikszentmihalyi, M. (1990). *Flow: The psychology of optimal experience.* New York: HarperCollins Publishers.

ABOUT THE AUTHOR

Clarissa Schilstra is a two-time cancer survivor. She was diagnosed with acute lymphoblastic leukemia for the first time when she was two and a half years old. She went through two and a half years of chemotherapy and survived. She led a happy and healthy life until June of 2007, when her cancer relapsed. So, she went through another two and a half years of chemotherapy, this time accompanied by radiation. She is now twenty-one years old and a senior at Duke University. Her passion is helping others cope with the ups and downs of life during and after cancer treatment. It is her goal to become a clinical psychologist after she graduates from Duke, and she would like to help improve the psychological care available to adolescents and young adults who have serious illnesses. You can read more about Clarissa on her website and blog at www.teen-cancer.com.

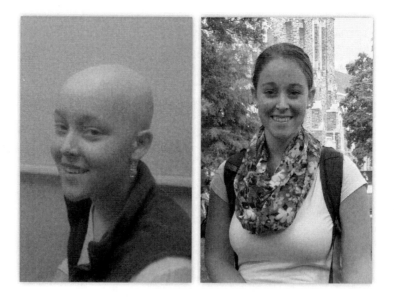